Radiology of RODENTS, RABBITS, AND FERRETS

An Atlas of Normal Anatomy and Positioning

Radiology of
RODENTS, RABBITS, AND FERRETS

An Atlas of Normal Anatomy and Positioning

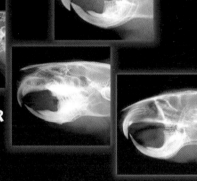
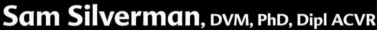
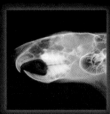

Sam Silverman, DVM, PhD, Dipl ACVR

Clinical Professor
Department of Surgery and Radiological Sciences
School of Veterinary Medicine
University of California, Davis
Davis, California

Lisa A. Tell, DVM, Dipl ABVP (Avian), ACZM

Professor
Department of Medicine and Epidemiology
School of Veterinary Medicine
University of California, Davis
Davis, California

RADIOGRAPHIC and TECHNICAL ASSISTANCE

Jody Nugent-Deal
Registered Veterinary Technician
Companion Avian and Exotic Pet Medicine Service
Veterinary Medical Teaching Hospital
University of California, Davis
Davis, California

Kristina Palmer-Holtry
Registered Veterinary Technician
Companion Avian and Exotic Pet Medicine Service
Veterinary Medical Teaching Hospital
University of California, Davis
Davis, California

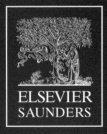

ELSEVIER
SAUNDERS

ELSEVIER
SAUNDERS

11830 Westline Industrial Drive
St. Louis, Missouri 63146

NOTICE

Veterinary Medicine is an ever-changing field. Standard safety precautions must be followed, but as
new research and clinical experience broaden our knowledge, changes in treatment and drug therapy
may become necessary or appropriate. Readers are advised to check the most current product infor-
mation provided by the manufacturer of each drug to be administered to verify the recommended
dose, the method and duration of administration, and contraindications. It is the responsibility of the
licensed prescriber, relying on experience and knowledge of the patient, to determine dosages and the
best treatment for each individual patient. Neither the publisher nor the authors assume any liability
for any injury and/or damage to persons or property arising from this publication.

International Standard Book Number 0-7216-9789-5

Acquisitions Editor: Anthony J. Winkel
Developmental Editor: Jolynn Gower
Publishing Services Manager: John Rogers
Senior Project Manager: Beth Hayes
Designer: Kathi Gosche
Cover Designer: Jyotika Shroff

Printed in the United States of America

Last digit is the print number: 9 8 7 6 5 4 3 2 1

*This book is dedicated to the veterinary clinicians, technicians,
and students who have helped to advance the medical care of our furred,
feathered, and scaled companions.*

SS and LT

*I dedicate this book to my parents, William and Bette Tell, and sister, Lee Ann Hughes,
who have provided me with unconditional love, support, and inspiration and enocouraged me
to follow my passion for veterinary medicine. I would also like to dedicate this book to
my husband, Don Preisler, children, Nicholas and Alexander Preisler, and mother-in-law,
Dawn Preisler, as they are a constant source of love and happiness and my life would not be
complete without them.*

LT

ACKNOWLEDGMENTS

The untiring efforts of many individuals made this atlas a reality. Hundreds of radiographic images were produced by Jody Nugent-Deal and Kristina Palmer-Holtry. Candi Stafford and Michelle Santoro provided technical advice and assistance to optimize image quality and develop radiographic protocols. Bob Smith was our technical liaison with the 3M Corporation. Jason Peters and Richard Larson developed the computed tomography techniques for acquiring thorough alternative imaging studies. Francesca Angelesco, John Gardiner, and Kathy West had exceptional artistic talents and technical skills. The attention to detail and resourcefulness of the aforementioned individuals resulted in production of quality images that serve as the basis of this text.

The animals imaged were integral to this text's creation. They were housed and maintained in compliance with the Animal Welfare Act and the Guidelines for the Care and Use of Laboratory Animals. All radiographic and alternative imaging procedures were performed according to an approved animal care and use committee protocol. We are indebted to the individuals who cared for these animals and provided permanent homes for them when imaging was completed.

The diagnostic images created for this text were catalogued, digitized, and reproduced by a technical support staff consisting of Jamie Ina, Andrea Pomposo, and Jennifer Chow, DVM. They also provided extensive research and technical support to the authors. John Duval assisted with digitization of radiographic images and graciously provided access to image processing equipment. Ned Waters donated his personal time and efforts to help digitize images when scanners were being serviced.

Drs. Seth Wallack, Karen Rosenthal, James Morrissey, Donald Thrall, David Crossley, and Frank Verstraete reviewed the text and images for accuracy and content. Dr. Helen Diggs was an invaluable resource and helped with the anatomic drawings. The insight of these individuals greatly enhanced this atlas.

The concept of this atlas evolved because of the vision of Ray Kersey, former Executive Editor of Veterinary Medicine for Elsevier. His dedication to disseminating veterinary medical knowledge cannot be understated.

Dr. Anthony Winkel, Jolynn Gower, Beth Hayes, and Kathi Goshe of Elsevier provided invaluable assistance during the final production phase of this atlas. Their dedication, hard work, and guidance regarding technical and esthetic matters were crucial and greatly appreciated.

Production of this atlas entailed 3 years of work, and we would be remiss not to acknowledge the goodwill, support, and understanding of our families. Our spouses, Debrah Tom and Don Preisler, constantly provided support and encouraged us to continue even though there were many hours devoted to the creation of the atlas rather than family affairs. Debrah Tom never failed to say "Have Fun" and Don Preisler responded with "No Problem" when told of a weekend of work ahead. Alexander and Nicholas Preisler made many visits to the Veterinary Medical Teaching Hospital on weekends to say hello to their Mom and to bring the entire crew refreshments.

In closing, we would like to extend our appreciation to all of these individuals for their encouragement, efforts and sacrifices. We are indebted to them for their persistence and dedication.

SS and LT

PREFACE

The species included in this text historically have been vital in biomedical research, but are becoming increasingly popular as companion animals. Documentation of radiographic and alternative imaging findings associated with disease conditions of these species has expanded greatly. However, there is no single reference that provides normal radiographic and alternative imaging anatomy for these species as there is for dogs, cats, horses, and other domestic animals. Diagnostic studies of these species were previously interpreted based on clinical experience and extrapolated knowledge from other species.

The purpose of this atlas is to provide veterinary clinicians with normal radiographic images and alternative imaging studies. We hope this atlas increases the utilization and accuracy of diagnostic imaging of these species and enhances their medical care.

CONTENTS

DETAILED CONTENTS

CHAPTER • **4**

Syrian (Golden) Hamster *(Mesocricetus auratus)*   45

CHAPTER • **5**

Domestic Chinchilla *(Chinchilla lanigera)*   67

CHAPTER • 6

Domestic Guinea Pig *(Cavia porcellus)* 105

CHAPTER • **7**

Domestic Rabbit *(Oryctolagus cuniculus)*   **159**

CHAPTER • **8**

Domestic Ferret *(Mustela putorius)*   **231**

CHAPTER 1

Radiology Equipment and Positioning Techniques

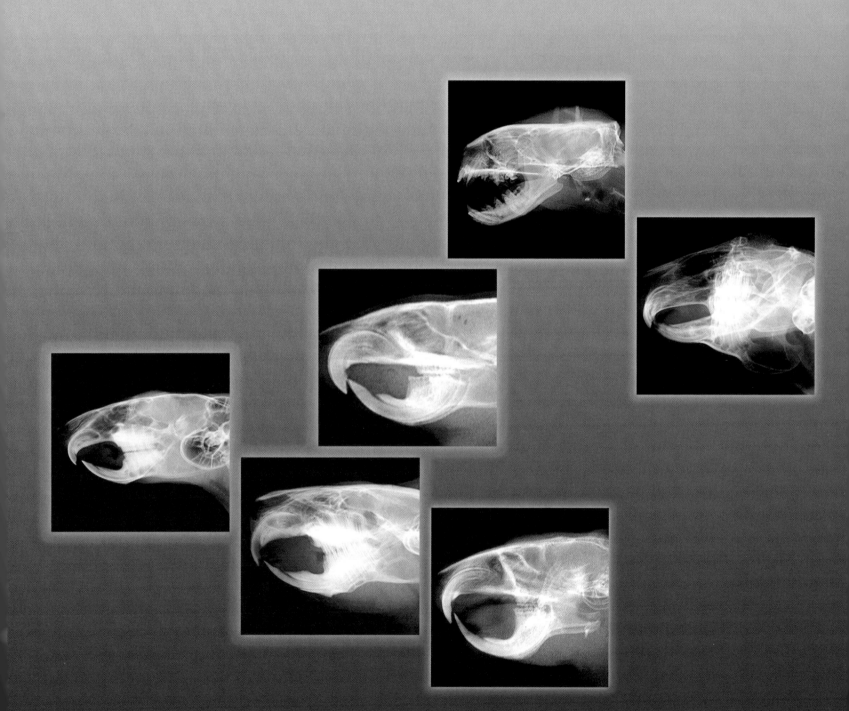

ANATOMIC REFERENCE

Images in this text were anatomically labeled to coincide with illustrations from *A Colour Atlas of the Anatomy of Small Laboratory Animals: Vols. I (Rabbit and Guinea Pig) and II (Rat, Mouse, and Golden Hamster)*, authored by P. Popesko, V. Rajtova, and J. Horak Wolfe (2002, WB Saunders, Philadelphia, Pa.).

Individual organs may not always be completely and clearly visualized on radiographs; therefore anatomic drawings have been provided as references for the rat, hamster, guinea pig, and rabbit. These anatomic drawings can be used as general guidelines. However, the location of abdominal organs may be affected by the animal's reproductive status and by distention of the digestive tract and urinary bladder. In addition, vertebral formulas for animals in this text may differ from those in other references because of individual variation.

RADIOGRAPHIC EQUIPMENT

The x-ray generator should be capable of 5.0 to 7.5 milliampere second (mAs) exposures, have a range of 40 to 100 kilovoltage peak (kVp), and be adjustable in 1- to 2-kVp increments. Rapid exposure times (i.e., 0.017 of a second and faster) should be possible to minimize patient motion artifact.

Most diagnostic x-ray tubes have small and large focal spots. Whenever possible, the small focal spot is selected because it produces radiographic images of superior detail. The disadvantage of the small focal spot is a lower milliampere capacity compared with the large focal spot, therefore requiring longer exposure times for equivalent milliampere second techniques. The small focal spot is also more prone to thermal damage associated with x-ray production. The height of the x-ray tube on the tube stand should be adjustable because it may be necessary to make small changes in the focal spot to film distance (FFD) to manipulate the exposure technique. The FFD used to produce the radiographic images in this text ranged from 38 inches (97 cm) to 40 inches (102 cm), except for the magnification studies. An Innovet Select 20kHz High Frequency Radiographic Machine (Summit Industries, Inc., Chicago, Ill. 60625) was used to produce the radiographic images in this book. Although the animals in this text are relatively small in body size compared to more traditional small animal veterinary patients (e.g., dogs and cats), an x-ray generator, an x-ray tube, and a tube stand with the aforementioned capabilities would offer maximal flexibility and are standard in most small animal veterinary clinics.

Asymetrix Detail Intensifying Screens (3M Animal Care Products, 3M Center, St. Paul, Minn. 55144-1000) and Ultra Detail Plus or SE+ radiographic film (3M Animal Care Products) were used to produce the radiographic images in this book. This film–screen combination produced a radiographic system speed of 100 to 350. Other film–screen combinations of similar speed and resolution could be used. Table 1-1 summarizes radiographic exposure factors used for creating this text's radiographic images using the table-top technique. These settings are intended to be guidelines and may require modification depending on the x-ray generator, film–screen combination, radiographic film processing, and patient size.

PATIENT POSITIONING

Imaging the animals included in this text can be challenging because of their resistance to restraint, small body size, relatively short extremities, and body conformation. It is often difficult to palpate anatomic landmarks because of thick subcutaneous adipose layers and luxuriant hair coats. Correct patient positioning is often achieved using visual anatomic landmarks rather than palpation.

Optimal image detail is obtained by performing studies on anesthetized or sedated patients. Anesthesia or sedation facilitates safe and accurate patient positioning and decreases patient motion artifact. All studies in this text were performed on anesthetized or sedated patients.

Important factors in patient positioning are symmetry and stabilization of the subject. Small pieces of radiolucent foam are occasionally used to aid positioning. Radiolucent paper masking tape is ideal for securing the patient's extremities. Weighted objects (e.g., sandbags) for extending and placing traction on the extremities are not as useful for the smaller patients because of their short limb length and the failure of weighted objects to conform to their extremities. Therefore smaller patients are secured directly on the cassette with tape. The extremities of larger patients may require more traction to prevent their limbs from obscuring the thorax and abdomen; therefore circumferentially wrapping their extremities with tape before the tape is secured to the cassette or table may be necessary. The following are brief descriptions of recommended positioning techniques.

POSITIONING TECHNIQUE FOR LATERAL RADIOGRAPHIC STUDIES OF THE WHOLE BODY, THORAX, AND ABDOMEN

The patient is placed on the cassette in lateral recumbency. The right lateral recumbent position is standard. The dependent limbs are fully extended, minimizing superimposition on the thorax and abdomen, and secured with tape to the cassette or table in a lateral position. The contralateral limbs are superimposed and similarly secured. The head is fixed in a straight lateral position by gently extending the neck and then securing the head and neck with tape onto the cassette or table. To optimize correct patient positioning, it is sometimes necessary to make minor positional adjustments to the head or extremities by placing small pieces of radiolucent foam under the nose or between the limbs. The tail is extended caudally and taped if necessary (Figures 1-1 to 1-3).

POSITIONING TECHNIQUES FOR VENTRODORSAL OR DORSOVENTRAL RADIOGRAPHIC STUDIES OF THE WHOLE BODY, THORAX, AND ABDOMEN

Obtaining ventrodorsal or dorsoventral radiographic images of the whole body, thorax, or abdomen is facilitated by the body conformation and flaccid muscle tone of these animals when they are anesthetized. For the ventrodorsal projection, the patient is placed on the cassette in dorsal recumbency. The pelvic limbs are symmetrically extended caudally, rotated slightly medially (adducted), and secured to the cassette or table if the legs extend beyond the cassette. The distal tips of the digits of both pelvic limbs are similarly positioned. The thoracic limbs are fully and symmetrically extended cranially, and the dorsal surfaces of the digits are placed on the cassette or table and secured with radiolucent tape. The head is placed in a straight ventrodorsal position and taped. A similar technique is used for the dorsoventral studies, but the patient is positioned in ventral recumbency. Gentle traction on the head and spine can be used to minimize rotation and other positioning artifacts (Figures 1-4 to 1-6).

POSITIONING TECHNIQUES FOR RADIOGRAPHIC STUDIES OF THORACIC AND PELVIC LIMBS

Radiographic images of entire thoracic and pelvic limbs are made with the patient in lateral or dorsal recumbency. Therefore radiographic images of the thoracic or pelvic limbs are mediolateral projections and ventrodorsal or dorsoventral projections, respectively. For a lateral radiographic study of the thoracic limb, the neck is extended dorsally to minimize superimposition of adjacent soft tissues on the extremity being examined. Positioning and securing limbs are similar to the methods described for the whole-body radiographic projections. Circumferential application of tape around the extremity is avoided because it induces limb rotation and may compress the digits, thereby reducing image detail. The x-ray beam is centered on the middle portion of the extremity, and the x-ray beam field includes the entire limb and a small portion of adjacent structures (Figures 1-7 to 1-9).

Table • 1-1

Radiographic exposure guidelines for rodents, rabbits, and ferrets using table-top technique and focal film distances of 40 inches (102 cm) for extremities and 38 inches (97 cm) for all other studies

Species	Approximate Body Size (g)	Radiographic Study	Film Screen System	mAs	kVp
Mouse	30	Whole body	**	7.5	48
		Skull	**	7.5	49
Hamster	150	Whole body	**	6.0	54
		Skull	**	7.5	52
Rat	300	Whole body	**	6.0	52
		Skull	**	6.0	52-53
Chinchilla	500	Whole body	***	5.0	44
		Skull	**	6.0	54-56
		Extremities	**	6.0	48-52
Guinea Pig	1200	Whole body	***	5.0	44
		Skull	**	7.5	54
		Extremities	**	6.0	48-52
Ferret	1200	Whole body	***	5.0	44
		Skull	**	6.0	54
		Extremities	**	6.0	48-52
Rabbit (small)	1200	Whole body	***	5.0	44
		Skull	**	7.5	54
		Extremities	**	6.0	48-52
Rabbit (medium)	2200	Whole body	***	5.0	45
		Skull	**	6.0	55
		Extremities	**	6.0-7.5	50-52
		Thorax	***	5.0	45
		Spine	***	7.5	47
		Pelvis	***	7.5	47
Rabbit (large)	4000	Whole body	***	5.0	46-48
		Skull	**	6.0	56-58
		Extremities	**	6.0-7.5	52-54
		Thorax	***	5.0	46
		Spine	***	7.5	48
		Pelvis	***	7.5	48

**3M (3M Animal Care Products, 3M Center, St. Paul Minn. 55144-1000) Asymmetrix Detail Intensifying Screen with SE+ radiographic film.
***3M (3M Animal Care Products, 3M Center, St. Paul Minn. 55144-1000) Asymmetrix Detail Intensifying Screen with Ultra Detail Plus radiographic film.

POSITIONING TECHNIQUES FOR RADIOGRAPHIC STUDIES OF EXTREMITIES

Positioning patients for lateral radiographic projections of the extremities is similar to that for the whole-limb examinations. For distal extremities to be in contact with the cassette and minimize rotation of the area of interest, additional strips of tape may be required. The tape is applied across the limb. Circumferential application of tape around the extremity is avoided because it induces limb rotation and compresses the digits, thereby reducing image detail. The contralateral limb should not be superimposed for these studies. The respective contralateral limb is circumferentially taped, and traction is applied to minimize superimposition on the limb being studied. The body is rotated appropriately to minimize superimposition of adjacent structures on the area of interest. Dorsal plane radiographic images of the thoracic limb distal to the antebrachiocarpal joint are termed *dorsopalmar* projections; in the pelvic limb dorsal plane radiographic images distal to the tarsocrural joint are termed *dorsoplantar* projections.

POSITIONING TECHNIQUES FOR RADIOGRAPHIC STUDIES OF THE HEAD

Radiographic studies of the head include lateral and dorsoventral radiographic projections and, when necessary, oblique views. For lateral and oblique projections, the patient is placed in a lateral recumbent position. For dorsoventral projections, the patient is positioned in ventral recumbency. Small wedges of radiolucent foam may be required for precise positioning

before the head is secured to the cassette. The oblique radiographic projections require rotation of 30 degrees or less off the straight lateral projection. Oblique projections are described by the point of entrance of the x-ray beam to the point of exit (Figures 1-10 to 1-11).

Magnification radiographic images of rodent and rabbit heads are included in this text. The principles of magnification radiography have been described in other veterinary radiology texts. In brief, the technique utilizes an ultrasmall focal spot x-ray tube and an increased object–film distance as compared to standard radiographs. The result is an enlarged image of the object being radiographed. These enlarged images are useful for critically examining small patients or body parts (Figure 1-12).

RADIOGRAPHIC CONTRAST STUDIES OF THE GASTROINTESTINAL TRACT

As a result of inherently poor tissue contrast of the animals represented in this text, special radiographic procedures can help to evaluate their digestive and urinary tracts. These studies can provide excellent anatomic detail, but evaluation of functional parameters can be compromised by the anesthesia or sedation used to acquire the images. Administration of contrast medium for gastrointestinal studies can be performed using a catheter-tipped syringe, a metal feeding tube, a soft flexible urinary catheter, or an esophageal tube. On occasion patients can be induced to swallow the contrast medium by

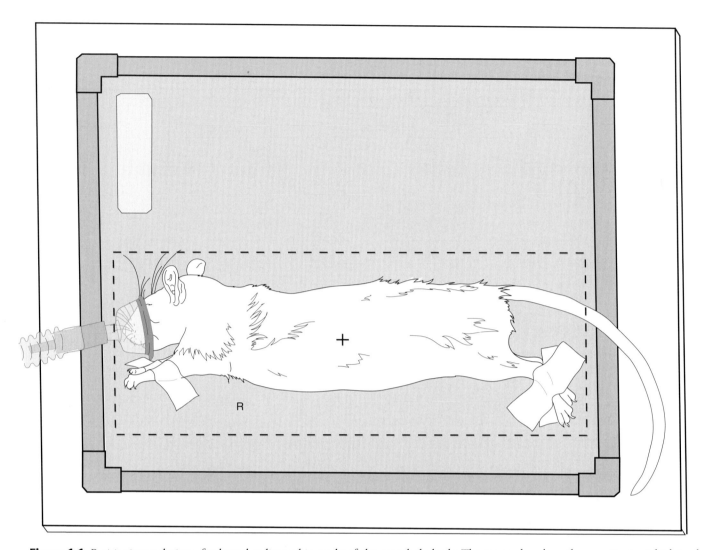

Figure 1-1 Positioning technique for lateral radiographic study of the rat whole body. The rat is placed on the cassette in right lateral recumbency. The thoracic limbs are secured to the cassette in full extension using radiolucent tape. The pelvic limbs are extended slightly caudally and taped. The x-ray beam *(+)* is centered on the middle portion of the body, and the x-ray beam field *(dotted lines)* includes the head and entire pelvis. (Drawing by Kathy West.)

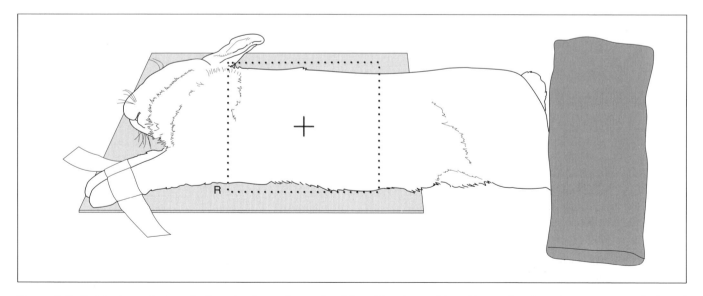

Figure 1-2 Positioning technique for lateral radiographic study of the rabbit thorax. The rabbit is placed on the cassette in right lateral recumbency. The thoracic limbs are secured to the cassette in full extension using radiolucent tape. Full extension of the thoracic limbs is required for optimal radiographic detail of the cranial thorax. The pelvic limbs are positioned using a sandbag (tape can be used instead of a sandbag). The neck is gently extended. The x-ray beam *(+)* is centered on the caudal border of the scapulae, and the x-ray beam field *(dotted lines)* includes the caudal cervical and cranial abdominal regions. The radiographic exposure is timed to coincide with peak inspiration.

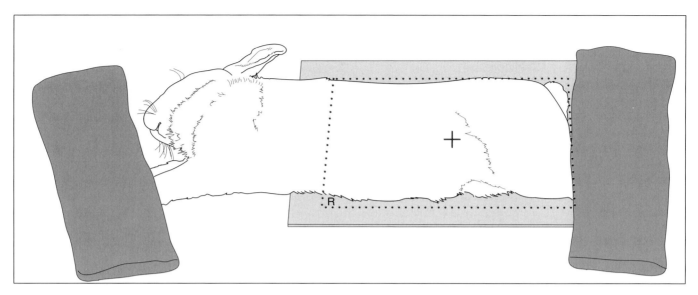

Figure 1-3 Positioning technique for lateral radiographic study of the rabbit abdomen. The rabbit is placed on the cassette in right lateral recumbency. The thoracic and pelvic limbs are extended and positioned using radiolucent tape or sandbags. The x-ray beam *(+)* is centered on the middle region of the abdomen, and the x-ray beam field *(dotted lines)* includes the caudal thorax and entire pelvis. The x-ray exposure is timed to coincide with the end of expiration.

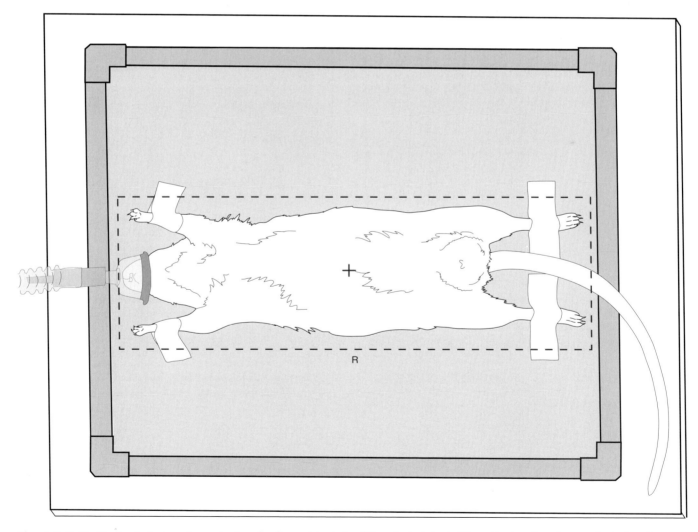

Figure 1-4 Positioning technique for ventrodorsal radiographic study of the rat whole body. The rat is placed on the cassette in dorsal recumbency. The thoracic and pelvic limbs are gently extended and secured to the cassette with tape. The x-ray beam *(+)* is centered on the midline at the thoracolumbar vertebral junction, and the x-ray beam field *(dotted lines)* includes the head and entire pelvis. (Drawing by Kathy West.)

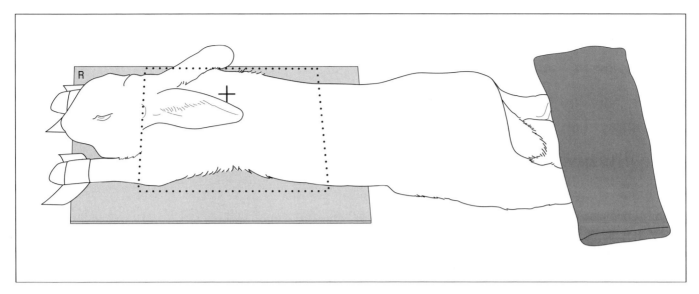

Figure 1-5 Positioning technique for dorsoventral radiographic study of the rabbit thorax. The rabbit is placed on the cassette in ventral recumbency. The thoracic limbs are extended and secured cranially and in close apposition to the skull rather than extended laterally. Cranial extension of the thoracic limbs minimizes superimposition of the scapulae and associated musculature on the cranial aspect of the thorax. The ears are positioned to minimize superimposition on the thoracic cavity. The x-ray beam *(+)* is centered on the midline of the middle portion of the thoracic vertebrae. The x-ray beam field *(dotted lines)* includes the caudal cervical and cranial abdominal regions. The radiographic exposure is timed to coincide with peak inspiration.

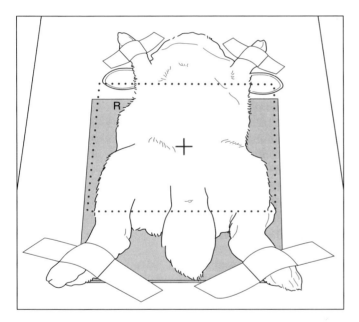

Figure 1-6 Positioning technique for ventrodorsal radiographic study of the rabbit abdomen. The rabbit is placed on the cassette in dorsal recumbency. The thoracic and pelvic limbs are gently extended and secured. The x-ray beam *(+)* is centered on the midline of the middle portion of the lumbar vertebral column. The x-ray beam field *(dotted lines)* includes the caudal thorax and entire pelvis. The x-ray exposure is timed to coincide with the end of expiration.

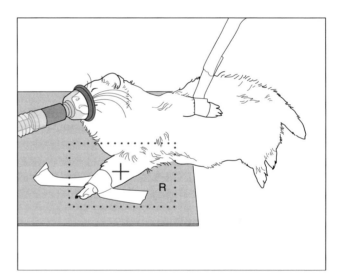

Figure 1-7 Positioning technique for lateral radiographic study of the ferret thoracic limb. The ferret is positioned in lateral recumbency so that the limb being radiographed is dependent. The thoracic limb is placed on the cassette and secured in the lateral position with radiolucent tape, and the contralateral limb is pulled caudally and dorsally to minimize superimposition of tissues. The x-ray beam *(+)* is centered on the elbow, and the x-ray beam field *(dotted lines)* includes the entire limb of interest.

slowly infusing it into the oral cavity through a catheter-tipped syringe or a metal feeding tube (avian gavage feeding tube) before anesthesia. In most instances the contrast medium is administered via an esophageal tube while the patient is anesthetized. Soft flexible urinary catheters or stomach tubes are preferred for esophageal or gastric administration, although rigid metal feeding tubes (avian gavage feeding tube) also can be used to dose nonanesthetized patients depending on the administrator's skill level. If a metal feeding tube is used, the ball-tipped orifice is placed in the

oral diastoma. Contrast medium is slowly infused as the patient swallows. The recommended volume of positive contrast medium for gastrointestinal procedures is approximately 2% of the body weight (2 ml of contrast medium/100 g of body weight). A suspension of micropulverized barium sulfate (60% weight/volume) was used for the gastrointestinal studies in this text.

In species with a relatively simple digestive system (e.g., mice, rats, and ferrets), double contrast gastrointestinal studies can be performed to provide superior detail of the mucosal

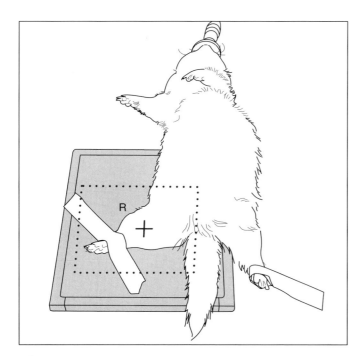

Figure 1-8 Positioning technique for lateral radiographic study of the ferret pelvic limb. The patient is positioned in lateral recumbency. The pelvic limb is placed on the cassette and secured in the lateral position with radiolucent tape. The contralateral limb is pulled caudally and abducted to minimize superimposition of soft tissues. The x-ray beam *(+)* is centered on the region of the stifle joint, and the x-ray beam field *(dotted lines)* includes the entire limb of interest.

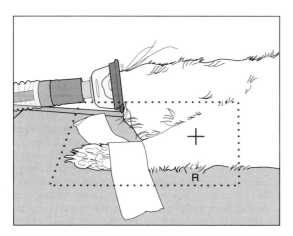

Figure 1-9 Positioning technique for ventrodorsal radiographic study of the ferret thoracic limb. The patient is placed in dorsal recumbency, but slightly rotated to the opposite side to minimize superimposition of soft tissues. The thoracic limb is placed on the cassette and secured in a ventrodorsal position with radiolucent tape. The x-ray beam *(+)* is centered on the region of the elbow joint, and the x-ray beam field *(dotted lines)* includes the entire limb.

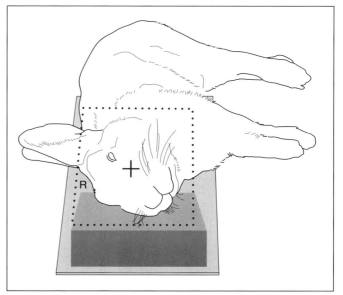

Figure 1-10 Positioning technique for lateral radiographic study of the rabbit head. The rabbit is placed in right lateral recumbency with the head resting on the cassette. A wedge-shaped piece of foam is placed under the rostral portion of the head so the sagittal plane is parallel to the top of the radiographic table. The legs are positioned symmetrically and the patient's body placed in a straight lateral position. If additional stabilization is necessary, radiolucent tape is used. The x-ray beam *(+)* is centered just rostral and ventral to the eye, and the x-ray beam field *(dotted lines)* extends to the cervical region.

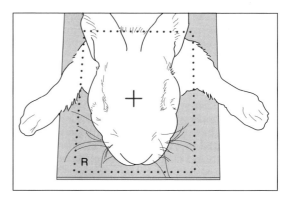

Figure 1-11 Positioning technique for dorsoventral radiographic study of the rabbit head. The patient is positioned in ventral recumbency with the mandible resting on the cassette. The thoracic limbs are extended cranially and laterally approximately 45 degrees to the long axis of the body to minimize superimposition on the head. The x-ray beam *(+)* is centered between the eyes on the midline, and the x-ray beam field *(dotted lines)* includes the entire head and extends to the region of the cervical vertebrae.

surfaces and to assess distensibility of the digestive tract. Double contrast gastrointestinal studies are performed under general anesthesia to minimize patient discomfort and obtain optimal distention of the digestive tract. Positive contrast medium (60% weight/volume barium sulfate) is first administered via a gastric tube. The volume administered is usually ¼ to ½ the calculated volume for positive contrast studies. Following barium sulfate administration, the stomach is distended with room air using the same gastric tube. The volume administered is usually 100% to 200% of the volume

of positive contrast medium administered for single contrast gastrointestinal studies. Complete gastric distention is desired. Double contrast studies should be performed with caution in patients with gastric tympany or potential gastrointestinal obstruction. If the stomach remains severely distended with gas after the last radiograph is made, the residual gastric gas should be evacuated by passing a gastric tube.

Colonic radiographic studies (barium enema) require retrograde infusion of contrast medium into the colon. Soft flexible catheters are usually sufficient. A suspension of

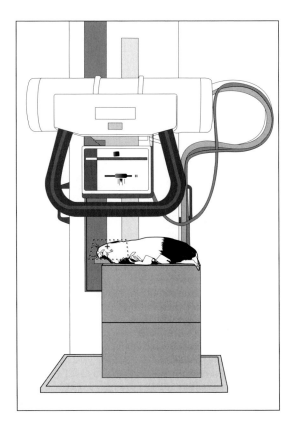

Figure 1-12 Table-top technique for a laterolateral magnification radiographic study of the guinea pig head. The cassette is placed on the top of the radiology table. The object–film distance (OFD) is increased by elevating the patient above the cassette with radiolucent foam sponge. The focal–film distance (FFD) is decreased by lowering the tube housing closer to the cassette. For the technique depicted in this illustration, the OFD is 12 inches (31 cm) and the FFD is 20 inches (51 cm). This technique resulted in a magnification factor of approximately 2.0.

micropulverized barium sulfate (60% weight/volume) is recommended. Precise dosing guidelines for retrograde colon studies have not been determined. The approximate colonic volume is estimated by evaluating the colon on survey radiographs. The length and diameter of the colon are the parameters used to approximate the colonic volume. One method of estimating the colonic volume is to superimpose a syringe barrel of similar diameter as the colon on the radiographs and follow the course of the colon through the abdomen. The number of syringe barrels necessary to course the entire length of the colon would be the estimated volume of barium used for the study. This estimation technique can be difficult

given the natural tortuous nature of the colon. Another method of volume calculation is to make radiographs during infusion of contrast medium, or if available the contrast medium infusion can be monitored fluoroscopically.

RADIOGRAPHIC CONTRAST STUDIES OF THE URINARY TRACT

Excretory urographic studies (rabbit and ferret) were performed after inserting a catheter into the cephalic vein and administering contrast medium intravenously. Abdominal compression was used to enhance visualization of the renal collecting system. Several layers of gauze sponge were applied to the ventral abdomen just cranial to the urinary bladder before compressing and wrapping the caudal abdomen with elastic bandage material. If urine production is low during the procedure, an intravenous diuretic can be administered after the contrast medium is injected. This may not be necessary in all patients.

Tomcat or small-diameter polyethylene catheters are used to administer contrast medium for retrograde cystography. Organic iodinated urographic contrast media with an iodine content of approximately 37% are acceptable. RenoCal-76 (66% diatrizoate meglumine and 10% diatrizoate sodium; Bracco Diagnostics, Princeton, NJ 08543) was used for the studies in this text. For double contrast procedures a small volume of positive contrast medium is first infused and then the urinary bladder is fully distended with gas. Although room air is commonly used, it does increase the potential for iatrogenic air embolism. Use of carbon dioxide gas (instead of room air) can prevent this complication. The volume of gas administered is determined by abdominal palpation during gas infusion. If the urinary bladder is prominently distended at the end of the study, contrast media and urine should be withdrawn through the catheter. A double contrast cystogram is particularly valuable in rabbits with a large amount of radiopaque urinary bladder debris.

MYELOGRAPHIC STUDIES

Performing myelography in guinea pigs, rabbits, and ferrets is similar to that described for dogs (*Textbook of Veterinary Diagnostic Radiology*, ed 4, Donald E. Thrall, editor, 2002, WB Saunders, Philadelphia, Pa., pp. 114-126). The anatomy of the spinal canal and cord of rodents and rabbits differs from that of feline and canine patients; therefore an anatomic text should be consulted. For obtaining survey radiographs of rabbits and guinea pigs, positioning the patient in ventral recumbency minimizes rotation. For the rabbit and guinea pig myelographic studies included in this text, contrast medium was injected under fluoroscopic guidance through a 27-gauge spinal needle. General anesthesia was used. As with any myelographic studies, anticonvulsant drug therapy should be considered.

CHAPTER 2

Laboratory Mouse *(Mus musculus)*

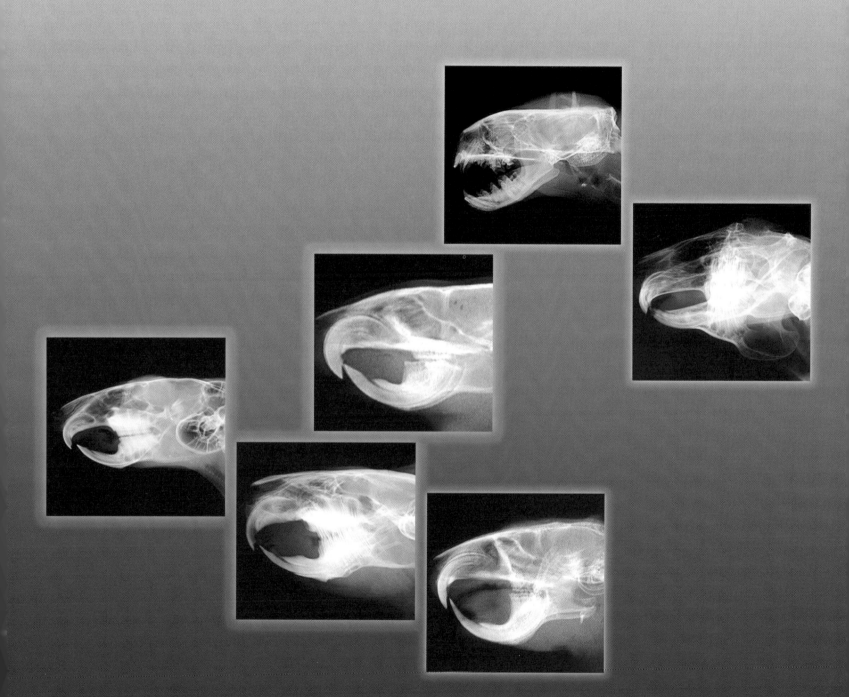

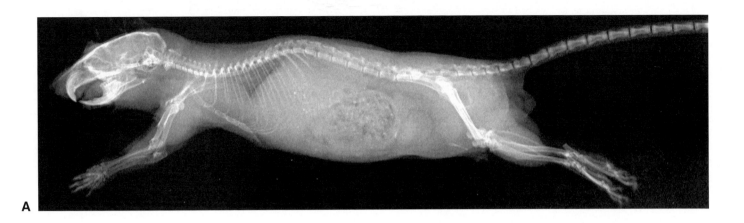

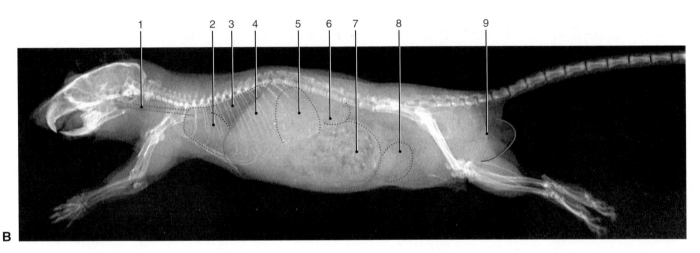

Figure 2-1, A and B
Type of animal: Mouse
Type of study: Viscera of thorax and abdomen
Projection: Laterolateral (right lateral recumbency)
Weight of animal: 27 g
Gender: Male
Reproductive status: Intact
Age: Adult

1. Trachea
2. Heart
3. Lung
4. Liver
5. Stomach
6. Kidney
7. Cecum
8. Urinary bladder
9. Scrotum

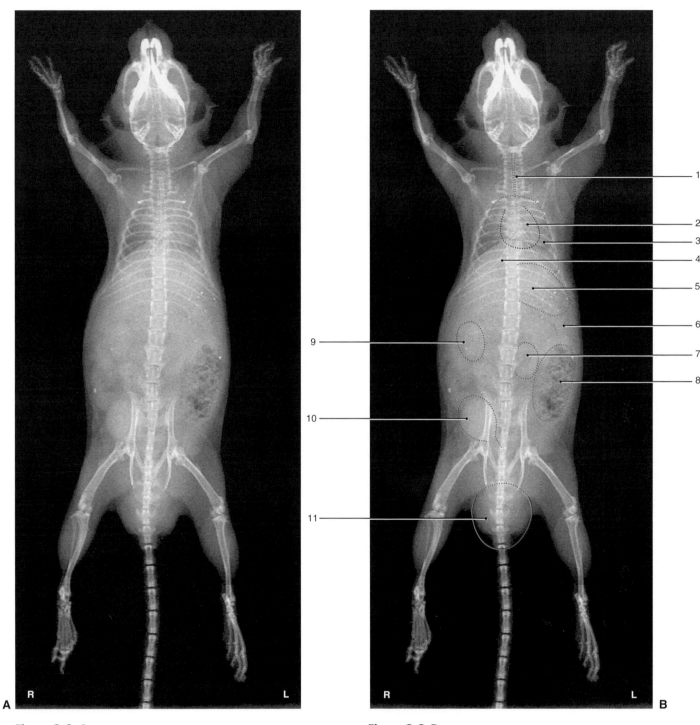

Figure 2-2, A
Type of animal: Mouse
Type of study: Viscera of thorax and abdomen
Projection: Ventrodorsal
Weight of animal: 27 g
Gender: Male
Reproductive status: Intact
Age: Adult

Figure 2-2, B
Type of animal: Mouse
Type of study: Viscera of thorax and abdomen
Projection: Ventrodorsal
Weight of animal: 27 g
Gender: Male
Reproductive status: Intact
Age: Adult

1. Trachea
2. Heart
3. Lung
4. Liver
5. Stomach
6. Spleen
7. Left kidney
8. Cecum
9. Right kidney
10. Urinary bladder
11. Scrotum

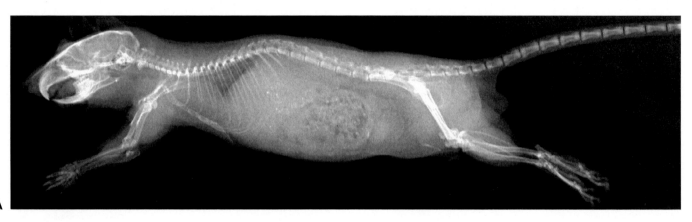

A

Figure 2-3, A
Type of animal: Mouse
Type of study: Whole body skeleton
Projection: Laterolateral (right lateral recumbency)
Weight of animal: 27 g
Gender: Male
Reproductive status: Intact
Age: Adult

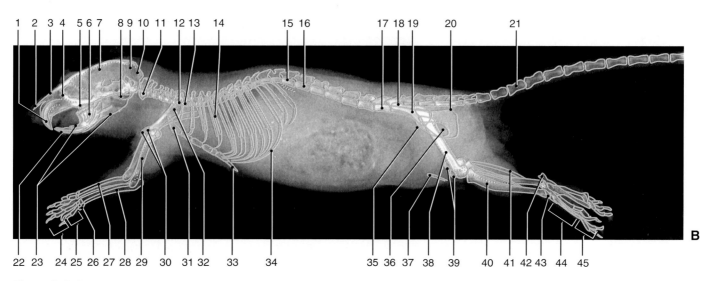

Figure 2-3, B
Type of animal: Mouse
Type of study: Whole body skeleton
Projection: Laterolateral (right lateral recumbency)
Weight of animal: 27 g
Gender: Male
Reproductive status: Intact
Age: Adult

1. Maxillary incisor tooth
2. Nasal bone
3. Incisive bone
4. Maxilla
5. Maxillary molar tooth
6. Mandibular molar tooth
7. Frontal bone
8. Tympanic bulla
9. Parietal bone
10. Occipital bone
11. Atlas
12. 7th cervical vertebra
13. 1st thoracic vertebra
14. 4th rib
15. 13th thoracic vertebra
16. 1st lumbar vertebra
17. 6th lumbar vertebra
18. Sacrum
19. Ilium
20. Ischium
21. Caudal vertebra
22. Mandibular incisor tooth
23. Mandible
24. Phalanges
25. Metacarpal bones
26. Carpal bone
27. Radius
28. Ulna
29. Humerus
30. Clavicles
31. Manubrium of sternum
32. Scapula
33. Xyphoid process
34. Costal cartilage
35. Pubis
36. Obturator foramen
37. Os penis
38. Femur
39. Patellae
40. Tibia
41. Fibula
42. Calcaneus
43. Tarsal bone
44. Metatarsal bones
45. Phalanges

Figure 2-4, A
Type of animal: Mouse
Type of study: Whole body skeleton
Projection: Ventrodorsal
Weight of animal: 27 g
Gender: Male
Reproductive status: Intact
Age: Adult

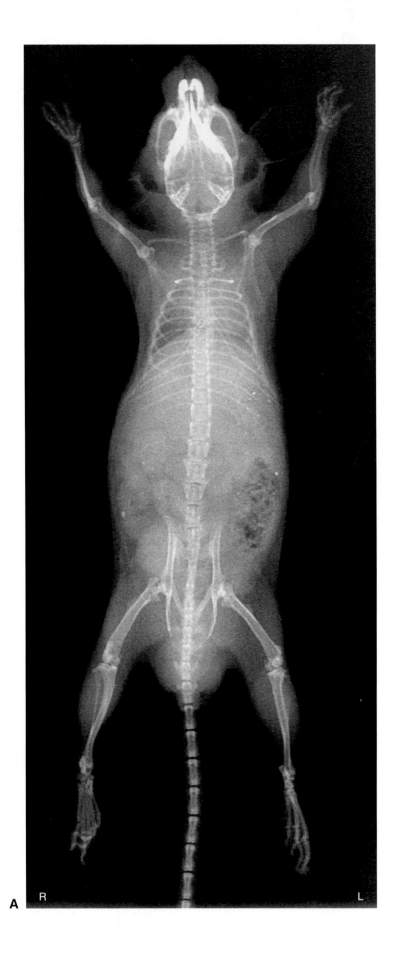

A

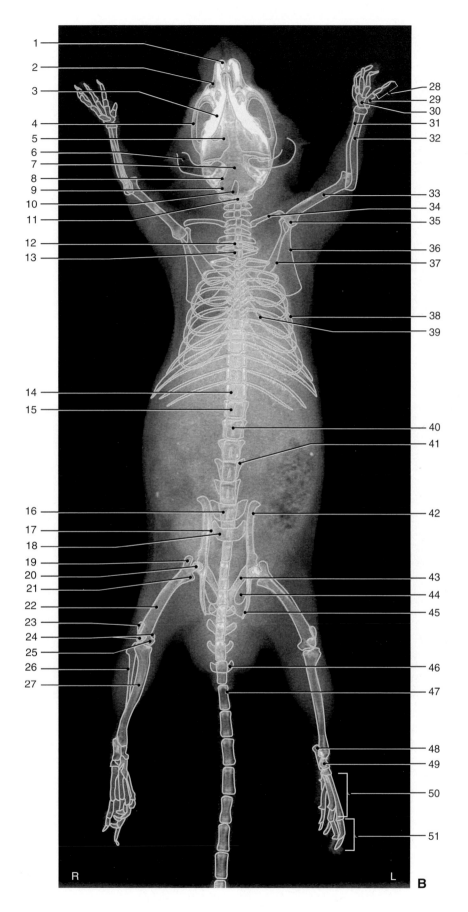

Figure 2-4, B
Type of animal: Mouse
Type of study: Whole body skeleton
Projection: Ventrodorsal
Weight of animal: 27 g
Gender: Male
Reproductive status: Intact
Age: Adult

1. Incisor tooth
2. Incisive bone
3. Mandible
4. Zygomatic bone
5. Frontal bone
6. Ear canal
7. Parietal bone
8. Tympanic bulla
9. Occipital bone
10. Foramen magnum
11. Atlas
12. 7th cervical vertebra
13. 1st thoracic vertebra
14. 13th thoracic vertebra
15. 1st lumbar vertebra
16. 6th lumbar vertebra
17. Sacroiliac joint
18. Sacrum
19. Greater trochanter of femur
20. Femoral head
21. Lesser trochanter of femur
22. Femur
23. Patella
24. Fabellae
25. Femoral condyle
26. Fibula
27. Tibia
28. Phalanges
29. Metacarpal bone
30. Carpal bone
31. Radius
32. Ulna
33. Humerus
34. Clavicle
35. Humeral head
36. Scapula
37. Spine of scapula
38. Rib
39. Costal cartilage
40. Spinous process of lumbar vertebra
41. Transverse process of lumbar vertebra
42. Ilium
43. Pubis
44. Obturator foramen
45. Ischium
46. Transverse process of caudal vertebra
47. Caudal vertebra
48. Calcaneus
49. Tarsal bone
50. Metatarsal bones
51. Phalanges

Figure 2-5, A
Type of animal: Mouse
Type of study: Head
Projection: Laterolateral
   (right lateral recumbency)
Weight of animal: 27 g
Gender: Male
Reproductive status: Intact
Age: Adult

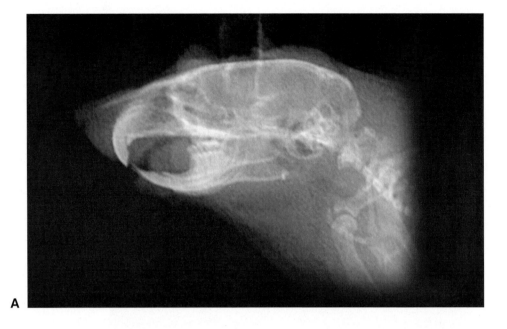

A

Figure 2-5, B
Type of animal: Mouse
Type of study: Head
Projection: Laterolateral
   (right lateral recumbency)
Weight of animal: 27 g
Gender: Male
Reproductive status: Intact
Age: Adult

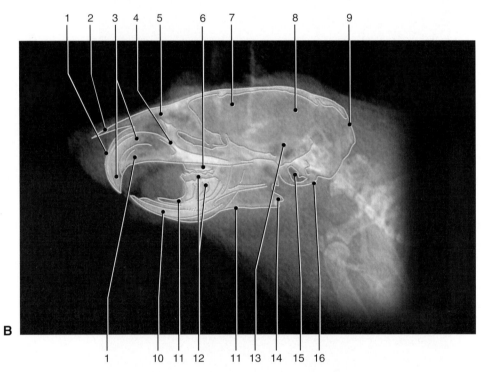

B

1. Incisive bone	9. Occipital bone
2. Nasal bone	10. Mandibular incisor tooth
3. Maxillary incisor tooth	11. Mandible
4. Zygomatic process of maxilla	12. Mandibular molar teeth
5. Maxilla	13. Temporal bone
6. Maxillary molar tooth	14. Angular process of mandible
7. Frontal bone	15. Tympanic cavity
8. Parietal bone	16. Tympanic bulla

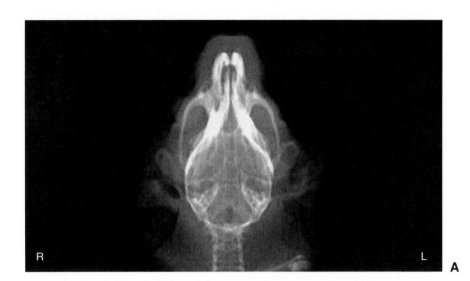

Figure 2-6, A
Type of animal: Mouse
Type of study: Head
Projection: Dorsoventral
Weight of animal: 27 g
Gender: Male
Reproductive status: Intact
Age: Adult

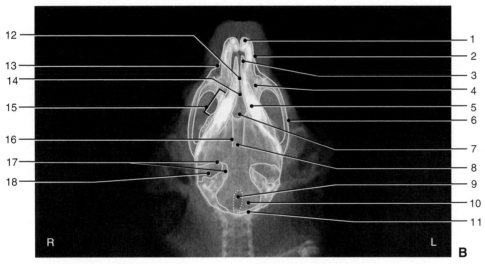

Figure 2-6, B
Type of animal: Mouse
Type of study: Head
Projection: Dorsoventral
Weight of animal: 27 g
Gender: Male
Reproductive status: Intact
Age: Adult

1. Maxillary incisor tooth
2. Incisive bone
3. Mandibular incisor tooth
4. Frontal bone
5. Mandible
6. Zygomatic bone
7. Palatine bone
8. Basisphenoidal bone
9. Foramen magnum
10. Occipital bone
11. Occipital condyle
12. Mandibular symphysis
13. Maxilla
14. Nasal cavity
15. Molar teeth
16. Pterygoid bone
17. Tympanic bulla
18. Tympanic cavity

CHAPTER 3

Norway Rat *(Rattus norvegicus)*

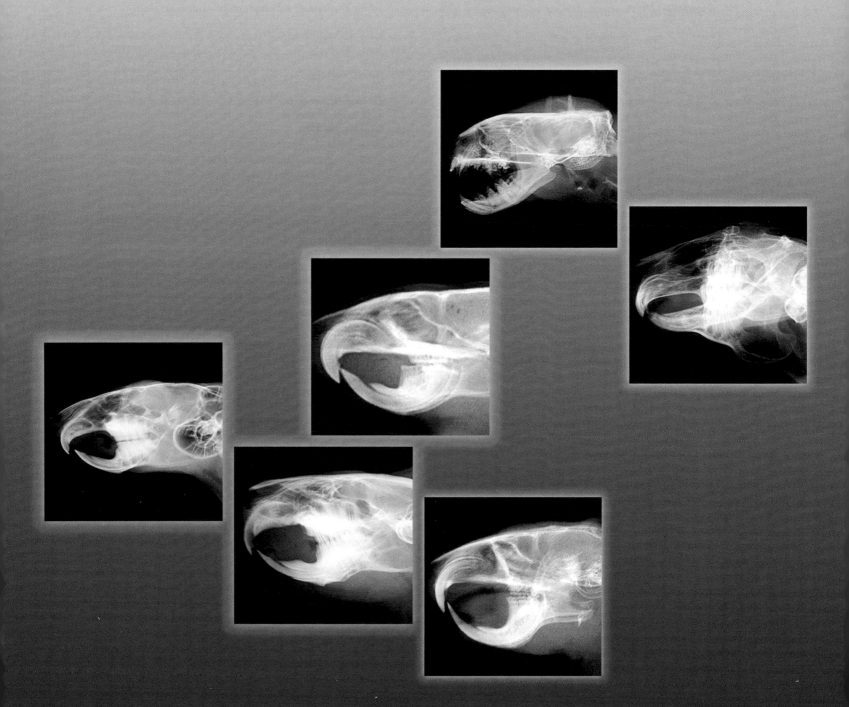

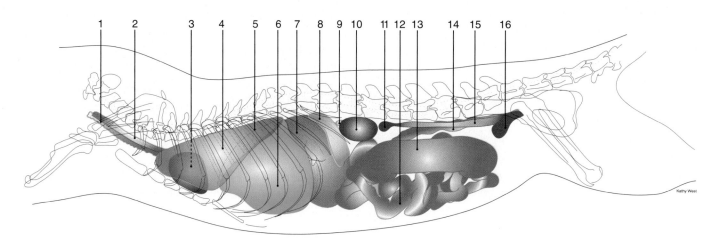

Figure 3-1, A Anatomic drawing (view of the left side) of viscera of the thorax and abdomen of an adult female rat.

1. Trachea
2. Esophagus
3. Heart
4. Lung
5. Diaphragm
6. Liver
7. Stomach
8. Spleen
9. Left adrenal gland
10. Left kidney
11. Left ovary
12. Small intestine
13. Cecum
14. Descending colon
15. Left horn of uterus
16. Urinary bladder

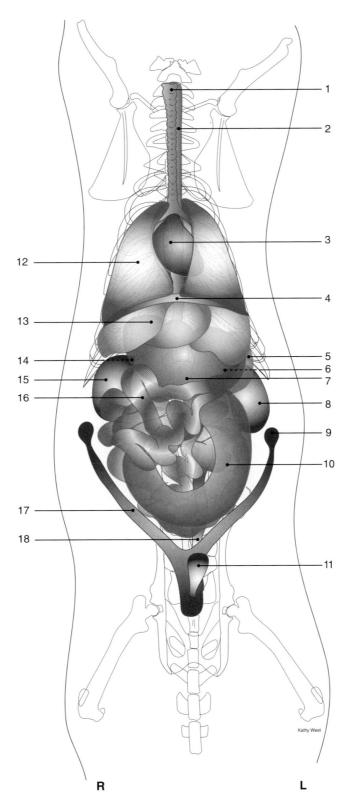

R   L

Figure 3-1, B Anatomic drawing (ventrodorsal view) of viscera of the thorax and abdomen of an adult female rat.

1. Trachea
2. Esophagus
3. Heart
4. Diaphragm
5. Spleen
6. Left adrenal gland
7. Stomach
8. Left kidney
9. Left ovary
10. Cecum
11. Urinary bladder
12. Lung
13. Liver
14. Right adrenal gland
15. Right kidney
16. Small intestine
17. Right horn of uterus
18. Descending colon

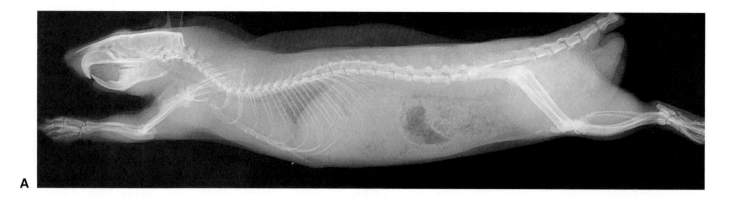

A

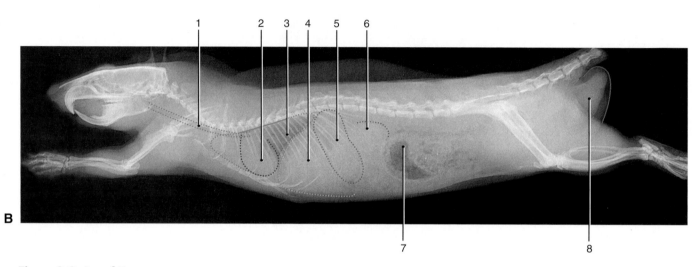

B

Figure 3-2, A and B
Type of animal: Rat
Type of study: Viscera of thorax and abdomen
Projection: Laterolateral (right lateral recumbency)
Weight of animal: 387 g
Gender: Male
Reproductive status: Intact
Age: Adult

1. Trachea
2. Heart
3. Lung
4. Liver
5. Stomach
6. Kidney
7. Cecum
8. Scrotum

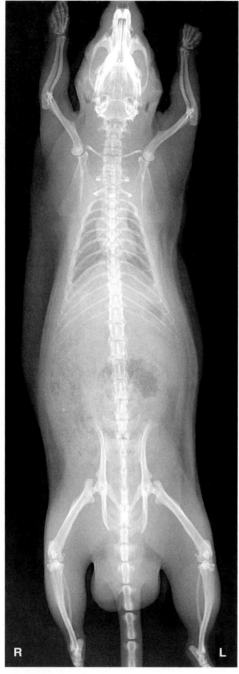

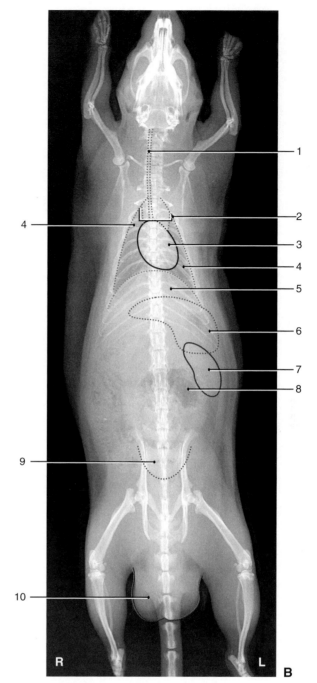

Figure 3-3, A
Type of animal: Rat
Type of study: Viscera of thorax and abdomen
Projection: Ventrodorsal
Weight of animal: 387 g
Gender: Male
Reproductive status: Intact
Age: Adult

Figure 3-3, B
Type of animal: Rat
Type of study: Viscera of thorax and abdomen
Projection: Ventrodorsal
Weight of animal: 387 g
Gender: Male
Reproductive status: Intact
Age: Adult

1. Trachea
2. Cranial mediastinum
3. Heart
4. Lung
5. Liver
6. Stomach
7. Left kidney
8. Cecum
9. Urinary bladder
10. Scrotum

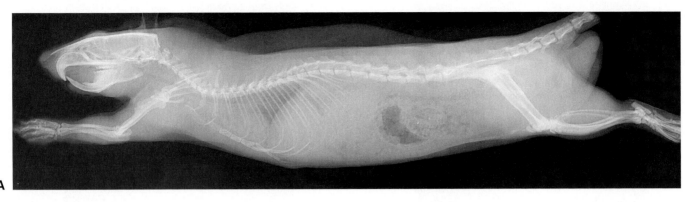

A

Figure 3-4, A
Type of animal: Rat
Type of study: Whole body skeleton
Projection: Laterolateral (right lateral recumbency)
Weight of animal: 387 g
Gender: Male
Reproductive status: Intact
Age: Adult

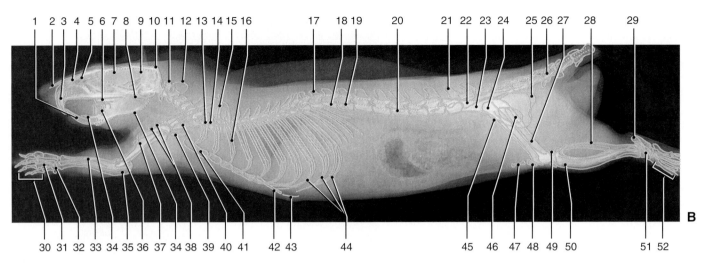

Figure 3-4, B
Type of animal: Rat
Type of study: Whole body skeleton
Projection: Laterolateral (right lateral recumbency)
Weight of animal: 387 g
Gender: Male
Reproductive status: Intact
Age: Adult

1. Mandibular incisor tooth
2. Nasal bone
3. Maxillary incisor tooth
4. Incisive bone
5. Maxilla
6. Maxillary molar tooth
7. Frontal bone
8. Tympanic bulla
9. Parietal bone
10. Occipital bone
11. Dorsal tubercle of atlas
12. Spinous process of axis
13. 7th cervical vertebra
14. 1st thoracic vertebra
15. Spinous process of 2nd thoracic vertebra
16. 3rd rib
17. Spinous process of thoracic vertebra
18. 13th thoracic vertebra
19. 1st lumbar vertebra
20. Transverse process of lumbar vertebra
21. Spinous process of 7th lumbar vertebra
22. Sacrum
23. Ilium
24. Femoral head
25. Ischium
26. Caudal vertebra
27. Femur
28. Fibula
29. Calcaneus
30. Phalanges
31. Metacarpal bone
32. Carpal bone
33. Radius
34. Mandible
35. Ulna
36. Mandibular molar tooth
37. Humerus
38. Clavicle
39. Suprahamate process
40. Scapula
41. Manubrium of sternum
42. 6th sternebra
43. Xyphoid process
44. Costal cartilages
45. Pubis
46. Obturator foramen
47. Os penis
48. Patella
49. Fabella
50. Tibia
51. Tarsal bone
52. Metatarsal bones

Figure 3-5, A
Type of animal: Rat
Type of study: Whole body skeleton
Projection: Ventrodorsal
Weight of animal: 387 g
Gender: Male
Reproductive status: Intact
Age: Adult

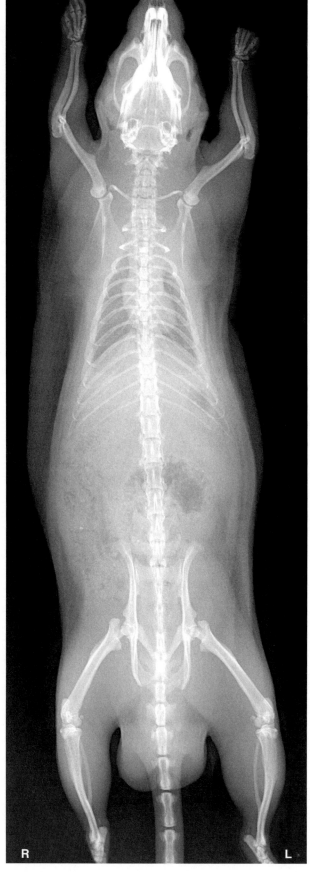

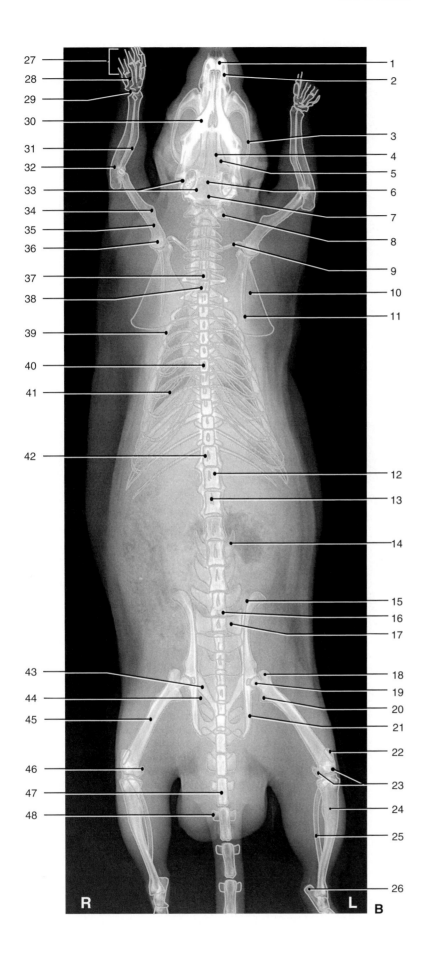

Figure 3-5, B
Type of animal: Rat
Type of study: Whole body skeleton
Projection: Ventrodorsal
Weight of animal: 387 g
Gender: Male
Reproductive status: Intact
Age: Adult

1. Maxillary incisor tooth
2. Incisive bone
3. Zygomatic bone
4. Pterygoid bone
5. Frontal bone
6. Parietal bone
7. Occipital bone
8. Transverse process of atlas
9. Clavicle
10. Scapula
11. Spine of scapula
12. 1st lumbar vertebra
13. Spinous process of lumbar vertebra
14. Transverse process of lumbar vertebra
15. Ilium
16. 7th lumbar vertebra
17. Sacrum
18. Greater trochanter of femur
19. Femoral head
20. Lesser trochanter of femur
21. Ischium
22. Patella
23. Femoral condyles
24. Tibia
25. Fibula
26. Calcaneus
27. Phalanges
28. Metacarpal bone
29. Carpal bone
30. Mandible
31. Radius
32. Ulna
33. Tympanic bulla
34. Deltoid tuberosity of humerus
35. Humerus
36. Humeral head
37. 7th cervical vertebra
38. 1st thoracic vertebra
39. Rib
40. Spinous process of thoracic vertebra
41. Costal cartilage
42. 13th thoracic vertebra
43. Pubis
44. Obturator foramen
45. Femur
46. Fabella
47. Caudal vertebra
48. Transverse process of caudal vertebra

Figure 3-6, A
Type of animal: Rat
Type of study: Head
Projection: Laterolateral
  (right lateral recumbency)
Weight of animal: 387 g
Gender: Female
Reproductive status: Intact
Age: 5 months

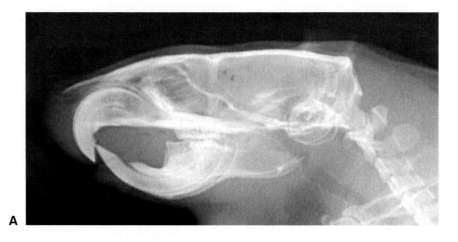

Figure 3-6, B
Type of animal: Rat
Type of study: Head
Projection: Laterolateral
  (right lateral recumbency)
Weight of animal: 387 g
Gender: Female
Reproductive status: Intact
Age: 5 months

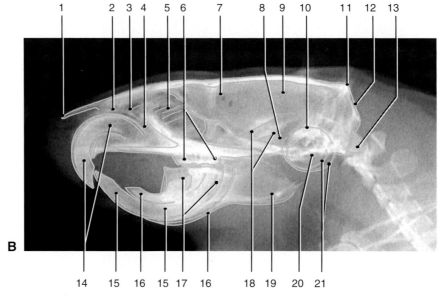

1. Nasal bone
2. Incisive bone
3. Nasoturbinates
4. Maxilla
5. Ethmoturbinates
6. Maxillary molar teeth
7. Frontal bone
8. Temporal bone
9. Parietal bone
10. Petrous part of temporal bone
11. External occipital protuberance
12. Occipital bone
13. Occipital condyle
14. Maxillary incisor tooth
15. Mandibular incisor tooth
16. Mandible
17. Mandibular molar teeth
18. Zygomatic process of temporal bone
19. Angular process of mandible
20. Tympanic cavity
21. Tympanic bullae

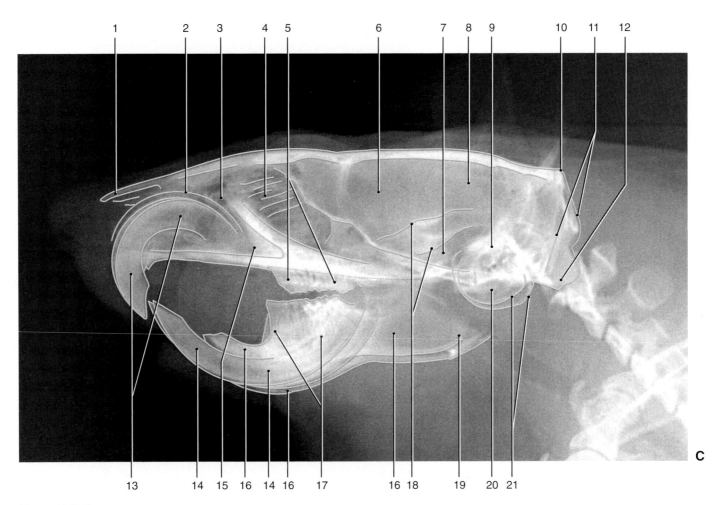

Figure 3-6, C
Type of animal: Rat
Type of study: Magnification study of head
Projection: Laterolateral (right lateral recumbency)
Weight of animal: 387 g
Gender: Female
Reproductive status: Intact
Age: 5 months

1. Nasal bone
2. Incisive bone
3. Nasal cavity
4. Ethmoturbinates
5. Maxillary molar teeth
6. Frontal bone
7. Temporal bone
8. Parietal bone
9. Petrous part of temporal bone
10. External occipital protuberance
11. Occipital bone
12. Occipital condyle
13. Maxillary incisor tooth
14. Mandibular incisor tooth
15. Maxilla
16. Mandible
17. Mandibular molar teeth
18. Zygomatic process of temporal bone
19. Angular process of mandible
20. Tympanic cavity
21. Tympanic bullae

Figure 3-7, A
Type of animal: Rat
Type of study: Head
Projection: Dorsoventral
Weight of animal: 387 g
Gender: Female
Reproductive status: Intact
Age: 5 months

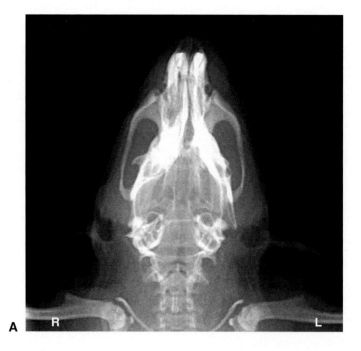

Figure 3-7, B
Type of animal: Rat
Type of study: Head
Projection: Dorsoventral
Weight of animal: 387 g
Gender: Female
Reproductive status: Intact
Age: 5 months

1. Nasal bone
2. Maxillary incisor tooth
3. Mandibular incisor tooth
4. Incisive bone
5. Infraorbital hiatus
6. Mandible
7. Zygomatic bone
8. Palatine bone
9. Pterygoid bone
10. Basisphenoidal bone
11. Tympanic bulla
12. Angular process of mandible
13. Petrous part of temporal bone
14. Parietal bone
15. Occipital bone
16. Maxilla
17. Zygomatic process of maxilla
18. Nasal cavity
19. Coronoid process of mandible
20. Tympanic cavity
21. Ear canal
22. Paracondylar process of occipital bone

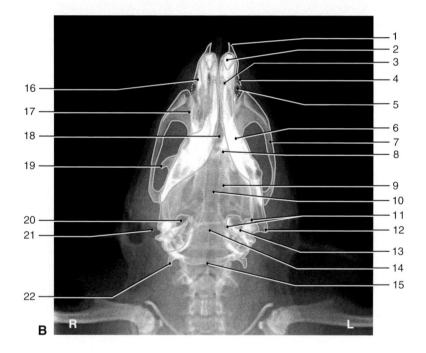

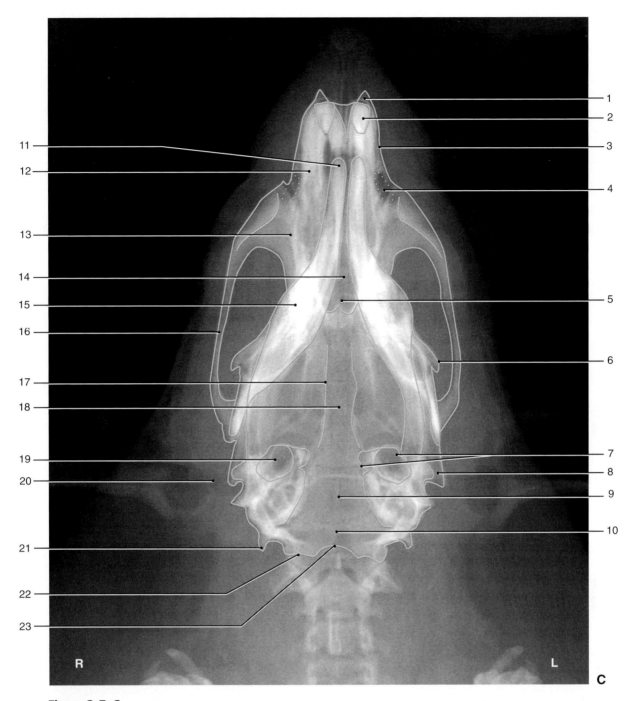

Figure 3-7, C
Type of animal: Rat
Type of study: Magnification study of head
Projection: Dorsoventral
Weight of animal: 387 g
Gender: Female
Reproductive status: Intact
Age: 5 months

1. Nasal bone
2. Maxillary incisor tooth
3. Incisive bone
4. Infraorbital hiatus
5. Palatine bone
6. Coronoid process of mandible
7. Tympanic bulla
8. Angular process of mandible
9. Parietal bone
10. Occipital bone
11. Mandibular incisor tooth
12. Maxilla
13. Zygomatic process of maxilla
14. Nasal cavity
15. Mandible
16. Zygomatic bone
17. Pterygoid bone
18. Basisphenoidal bone
19. Tympanic cavity
20. Ear canal
21. Paracondylar process of occipital bone
22. Occipital condyle
23. Foramen magnum

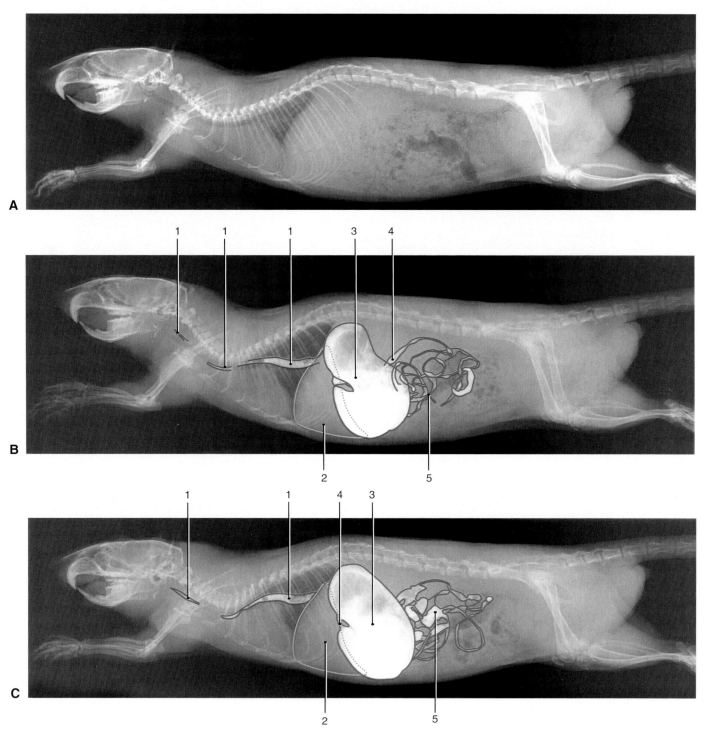

Figure 3-8, A-G

Type of animal: Rat

Type of study: Gastrointestinal positive contrast study

Contrast medium: Barium sulfate suspension (Novopaque 60% w/v; Lafayette Pharmaceutical, Inc., Lafayette, Ind.) 5 ml administered via esophageal gavage

Projection: Laterolateral (right lateral recumbency)

Weight of animal: 224 g

Gender: Male

Reproductive status: Intact

Age: Adult

1. Esophagus
2. Liver
3. Stomach
4. Duodenum
5. Small intestine
6. Ileum
7. Cecum
8. Colon
9. Rectum

Image	Time (hr)
A	Survey
B	0.25
C	0.50

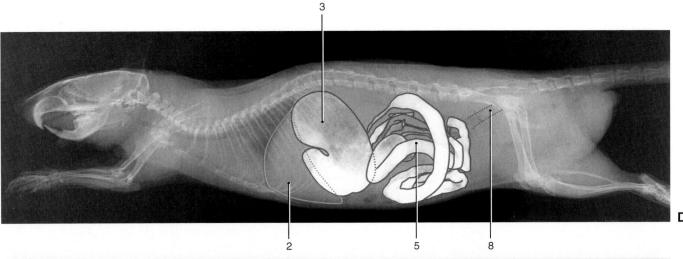

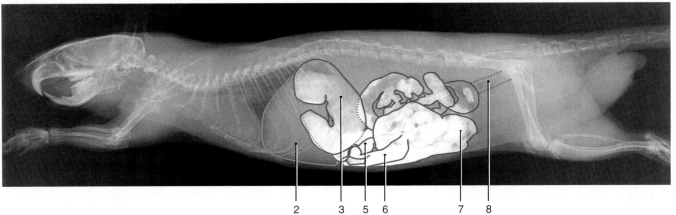

Figure 3-8, A-G—cont'd
Type of animal: Rat
Type of study: Gastrointestinal positive contrast study
Contrast medium: Barium sulfate suspension (Novopaque 60% w/v; Lafayette Pharmaceutical, Inc., Lafayette, Ind.) 5 ml administered via esophageal gavage
Projection: Laterolateral (right lateral recumbency)
Weight of animal: 224 g
Gender: Male
Reproductive status: Intact
Age: Adult

1. Esophagus
2. Liver
3. Stomach
4. Duodenum
5. Small intestine
6. Ileum
7. Cecum
8. Colon
9. Rectum

Image	Time (hr)
D	2.75
E	5.25

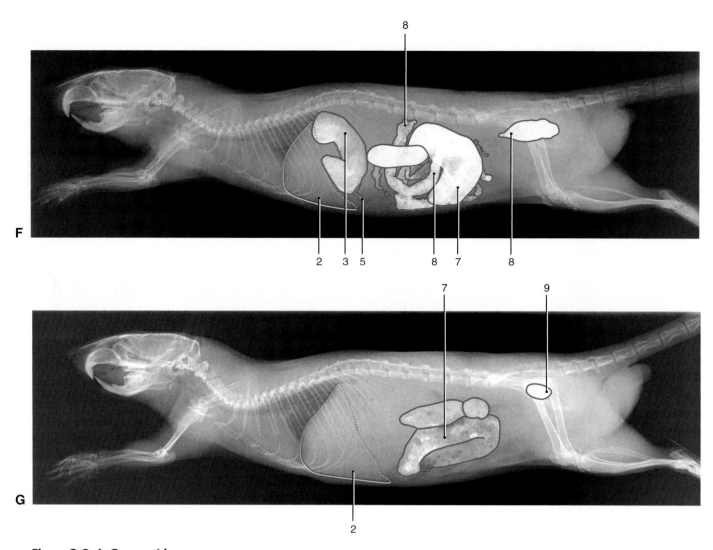

Figure 3-8, A-G—cont'd
Type of animal: Rat
Type of study: Gastrointestinal positive contrast study
Contrast medium: Barium sulfate suspension (Novopaque
    60% w/v; Lafayette Pharmaceutical, Inc., Lafayette, Ind.)
    5 ml administered via esophageal gavage
Projection: Laterolateral (right lateral recumbency)
Weight of animal: 224 g
Gender: Male
Reproductive status: Intact
Age: Adult

1. Esophagus
2. Liver
3. Stomach
4. Duodenum
5. Small intestine
6. Ileum
7. Cecum
8. Colon
9. Rectum

Image	Time (hr)
F	8.25
G	22.00

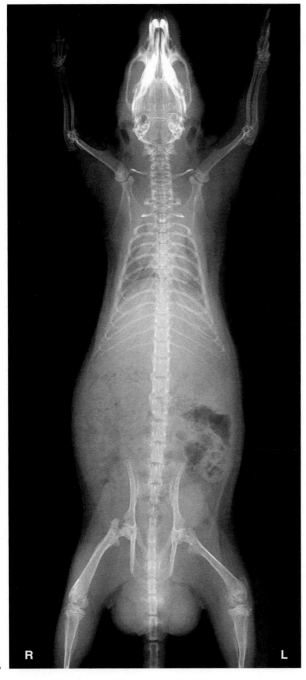

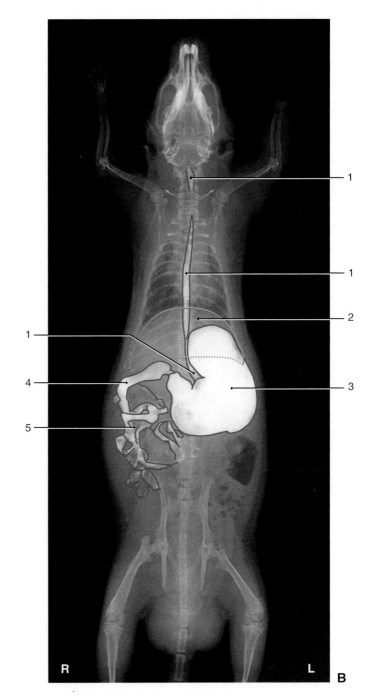

Figure 3-9, A-G
Type of animal: Rat
Type of study: Gastrointestinal positive contrast study
Contrast medium: Barium sulfate suspension (Novopaque
    60% w/v; Lafayette Pharmaceutical, Inc., Lafayette, Ind.)
    5 ml administered via esophageal gavage
Projection: Ventrodorsal
Weight of animal: 224 g
Gender: Male
Reproductive status: Intact
Age: Adult

1. Esophagus
2. Liver
3. Stomach
4. Duodenum
5. Small intestine
6. Ileum
7. Cecum
8. Colon
9. Rectum

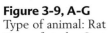

Image	Time (hr)
A	Survey
B	0.25

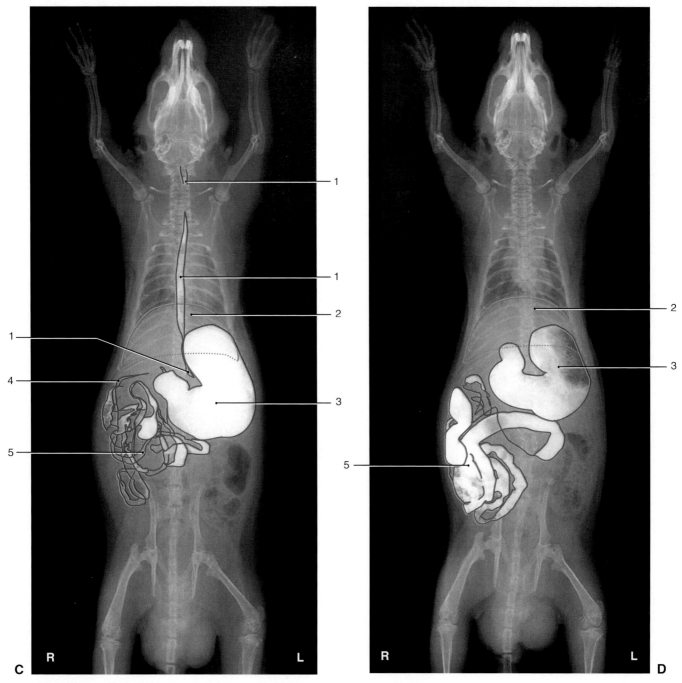

Figure 3-9, A-G—cont'd
Type of animal: Rat
Type of study: Gastrointestinal positive contrast study
Contrast medium: Barium sulfate suspension (Novopaque 60% w/v; Lafayette Pharmaceutical, Inc., Lafayette, Ind.) 5 ml administered via esophageal gavage
Projection: Ventrodorsal
Weight of animal: 224 g
Gender: Male
Reproductive status: Intact
Age: Adult

1. Esophagus
2. Liver
3. Stomach
4. Duodenum
5. Small intestine
6. Ileum
7. Cecum
8. Colon
9. Rectum

Image	Time (hr)
C	0.50
D	2.75

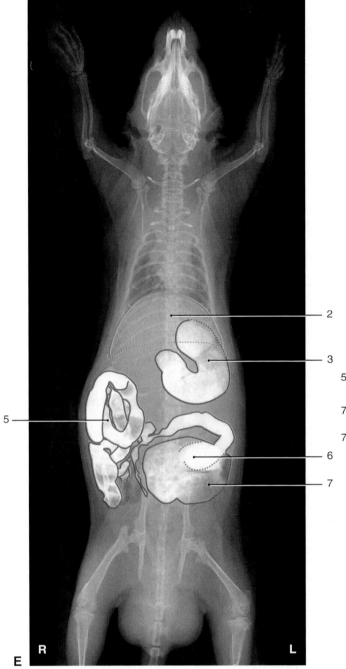

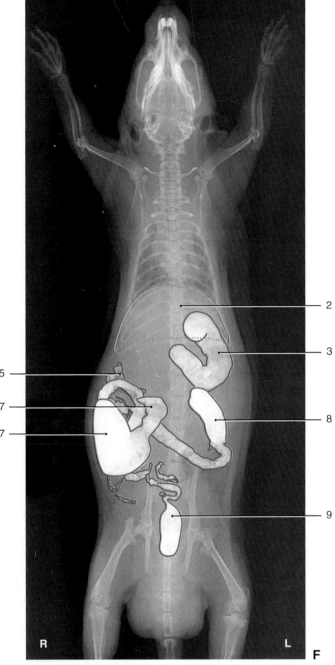

Figure 3-9, A-G—cont'd
Type of animal: Rat
Type of study: Gastrointestinal positive contrast study
Contrast medium: Barium sulfate suspension (Novopaque
  60% w/v; Lafayette Pharmaceutical, Inc., Lafayette, Ind.)
  5 ml administered via esophageal gavage
Projection: Ventrodorsal
Weight of animal: 224 g
Gender: Male
Reproductive status: Intact
Age: Adult

1. Esophagus
2. Liver
3. Stomach
4. Duodenum
5. Small intestine
6. Ileum
7. Cecum
8. Colon
9. Rectum

Image	Time (hr)
E	5.25
F	8.25

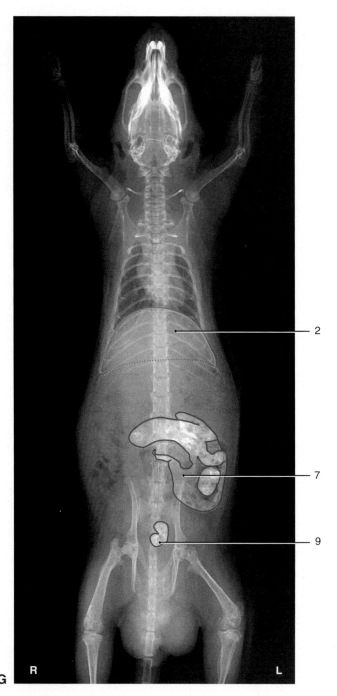

Figure 3-9, A-G—cont'd

Type of animal: Rat
Type of study: Gastrointestinal positive contrast study
Contrast medium: Barium sulfate suspension (Novopaque
    60% w/v; Lafayette Pharmaceutical, Inc., Lafayette, Ind.)
    5 ml administered via esophageal gavage
Projection: Ventrodorsal
Weight of animal: 224 g
Gender: Male
Reproductive status: Intact
Age: Adult

1. Esophagus
2. Liver
3. Stomach
4. Duodenum
5. Small intestine
6. Ileum
7. Cecum
8. Colon
9. Rectum

Image	Time (hr)
G	22.00

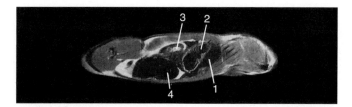

Figure 3-10 Longitudinal view of the body. (From Krinke GJ, editor: *The laboratory rat*, San Diego, 2000, Academic Press.)

1. Liver
2. Stomach
3. Left kidney
4. Cecum

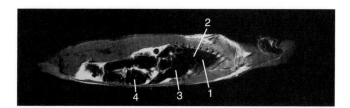

Figure 3-11 Longitudinal view of the body. (From Krinke GJ, editor: *The laboratory rat*, San Diego, 2000, Academic Press.)

1. Lung
2. Diaphragm
3. Liver
4. Cecum

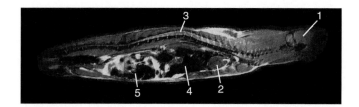

Figure 3-12 Longitudinal view of the body. (From Krinke GJ, editor: *The laboratory rat*, San Diego, 2000, Academic Press.)

1. Brain
2. Heart
3. Spinal cord
4. Liver
5. Intestinal tract

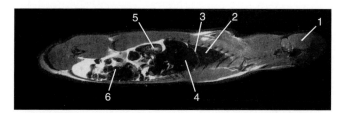

Figure 3-13 Longitudinal view of the body. (From Krinke GJ, editor: *The laboratory rat*, San Diego, 2000, Academic Press.)

1. Brain
2. Lung
3. Diaphragm
4. Liver
5. Right kidney
6. Intestinal tract

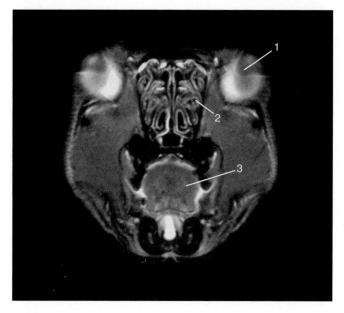

Figure 3-14 Transverse view of the head. (From Krinke GJ, editor: *The laboratory rat*, San Diego, 2000, Academic Press.)

1. Eye
2. Nasal cavity
3. Tongue

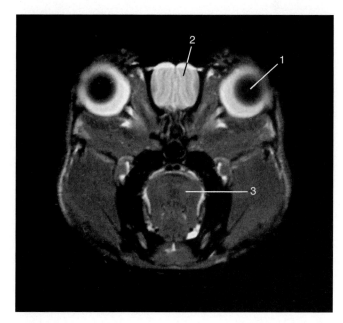

Figure 3-15 Transverse view of the head. (From Krinke GJ, editor: *The laboratory rat*, San Diego, 2000, Academic Press.)

1. Eye
2. Bulbus olfactorius
3. Tongue

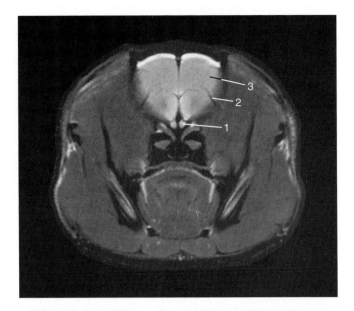

Figure 3-16 Transverse view of the head. (From Krinke GJ, editor: *The laboratory rat*, San Diego, 2000, Academic Press.)

1. Optic nerve
2. Fissura rhinalis
3. Frontal cerebral hemisphere

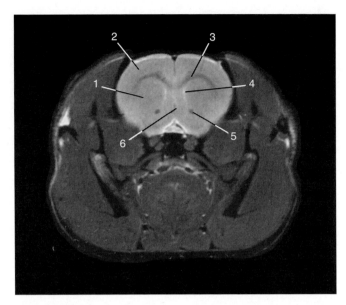

Figure 3-17 Transverse view of the head. (From Krinke GJ, editor: *The laboratory rat*, San Diego, 2000, Academic Press.)

1. Basal ganglia (caudatoputamen)
2. Frontal cortex
3. Corpus callosum
4. Lateral cerebral ventricle
5. Commissura anterior
6. Area parolfactoria

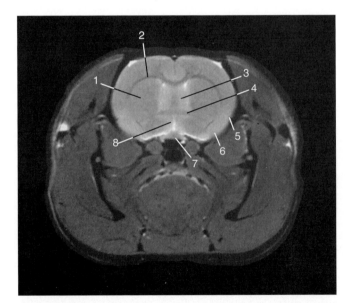

Figure 3-18 Transverse view of the head. (From Krinke GJ, editor: *The laboratory rat*, San Diego, 2000, Academic Press.)

1. Basal ganglia (caudatoputamen)
2. Corpus callosum
3. Septum
4. Commissura anterior
5. Fissura rhinalis
6. Cortex piriformis
7. Chiasma opticum
8. Area preoptica

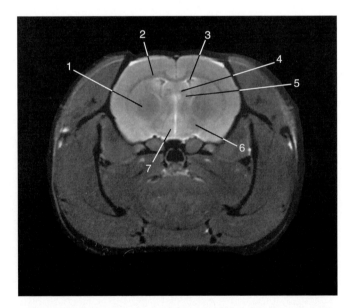

Figure 3-19 Transverse view of the head. (From Krinke GJ, editor: *The laboratory rat*, San Diego, 2000, Academic Press.)

1. Basal ganglia (caudatoputamen)
2. Corpus callosum
3. Lateral cerebral ventricle
4. Septum
5. Stria medullaris thalami
6. Fasciculus medialis telencephali
7. Anterior hypothalamus

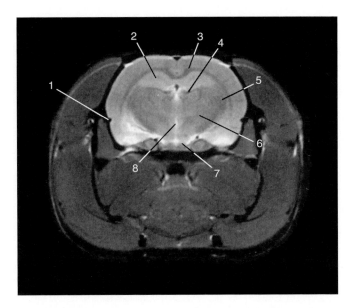

Figure 3-20 Transverse view of the head. (From Krinke GJ, editor: *The laboratory rat*, San Diego, 2000, Academic Press.)

1. Fissura rhinalis
2. Dorsal hippocampus
3. Corpus callosum
4. Stria medullaris thalami
5. Thalamus
6. Lemniscus medialis
7. Hypothalamus
8. Third cerebral ventricle

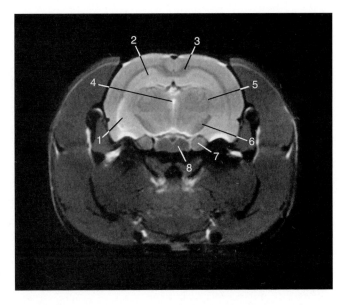

Figure 3-21 Transverse view of the head. (From Krinke GJ, editor: *The laboratory rat*, San Diego, 2000, Academic Press.)

1. Ventral hippocampus
2. Dorsal hippocampus
3. Corpus callosum
4. Third cerebral ventricle
5. Thalamus
6. Pedunculus cerebri
7. Trigeminal nerve
8. Pituitary gland

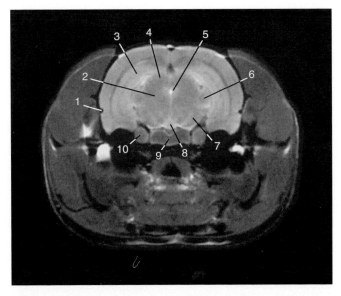

Figure 3-22 Transverse view of the head. (From Krinke GJ, editor: *The laboratory rat*, San Diego, 2000, Academic Press.)

1. Fissura rhinalis
2. Tegmentum mesencephali
3. Hippocampus
4. Colliculus superior
5. Substantia grisea centralis
6. Corpus geniculatum mediale
7. Pedunculus cerebri
8. Nucleus interpeduncularis
9. Pituitary gland
10. Trigeminal root

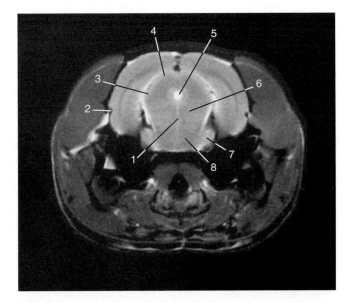

Figure 3-23 Transverse view of the head. (From Krinke GJ, editor: *The laboratory rat*, San Diego, 2000, Academic Press.)

1. Raphe
2. Fissura rhinalis
3. Colliculus inferior
4. Colliculus superior
5. Aqueductus cerebri
6. Formatio reticularis
7. Pedunculus cerebellaris medius and trigeminal root
8. Pons and tractus corticospinalis

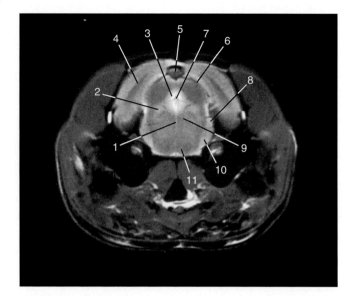

Figure 3-24 Transverse view of the head. (From Krinke GJ, editor: *The laboratory rat*, San Diego, 2000, Academic Press.)

1. Raphe
2. Pedunculus cerebellaris superior
3. Substantia grisea centralis
4. Occipital cortex
5. Pineal body
6. Colliculus inferior
7. Aqueductus cerebri
8. Pedunculus cerebellaris medius
9. Formatio reticularis
10. Spinal trigeminal root
11. Tractus corticospinalis

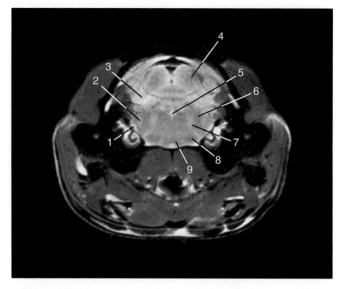

Figure 3-25 Transverse view of the head. (From Krinke GJ, editor: *The laboratory rat*, San Diego, 2000, Academic Press.)

1. Spinal trigeminal root
2. Trigeminal motor root
3. Cerebellar cortex
4. Colliculus inferior
5. Fourth cerebral ventricle
6. Trigeminal motor nucleus
7. Radix nervi facialis
8. Complexus olivae superioris
9. Corticospinal tract

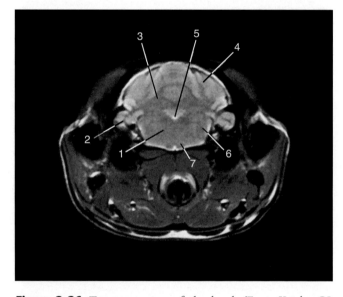

Figure 3-26 Transverse view of the head. (From Krinke GJ, editor: *The laboratory rat*, San Diego, 2000, Academic Press.)

1. Reticular nuclei
2. Paraflocculus
3. Deep cerebellar nuclei
4. Cerebellar cortex
5. Fourth cerebral ventricle
6. Spinal trigeminal tract and nucleus
7. Corticospinal tract

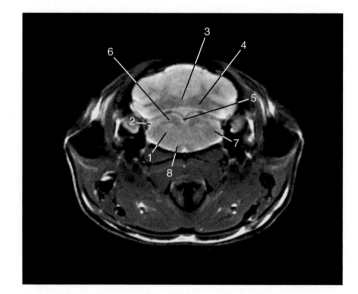

Figure 3-27 Transverse view of the head. (From Krinke GJ, editor: *The laboratory rat*, San Diego, 2000, Academic Press.)

1. Reticular nuclei
2. Spinocerebellar tract
3. Cerebellar cortex
4. Deep cerebellar nuclei
5. Fourth cerebral ventricle
6. Vestibular nuclei
7. Spinal trigeminal tract and nucleus
8. Corticospinal tract

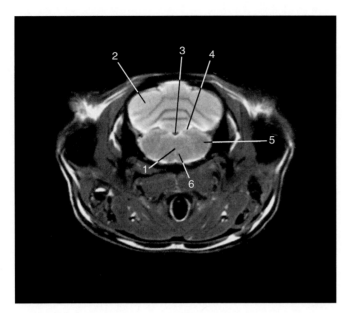

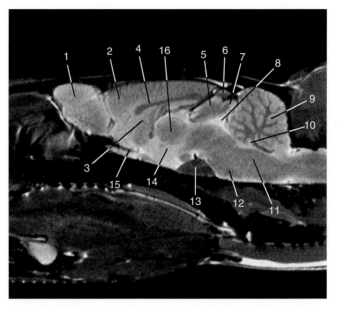

Figure 3-28 Transverse view of the head. (From Krinke GJ, editor: *The laboratory rat*, San Diego, 2000, Academic Press.)

1. Raphe
2. Cerebellar cortex
3. Fourth cerebral ventricle
4. Cuneate nucleus and fascicle
5. Spinal trigeminal root and nucleus
6. Corticospinal tract

Figure 3-29 Mid-longitudinal view of the head. (From Krinke GJ, editor: *The laboratory rat*, San Diego, 2000, Academic Press.)

1. Bulbus olfactorius
2. Cerebral cortex
3. Septum
4. Corpus callosum
5. Colliculus anterior
6. Pineal body
7. Colliculus posterior
8. Aqueduct
9. Cerebellum
10. Fourth cerebral ventricle
11. Medulla oblongata
12. Pons
13. Pituitary gland
14. Third cerebral ventricle
15. Optic nerve
16. Thalamus

CHAPTER 4

Syrian (Golden) Hamster *(Mesocricetus auratus)*

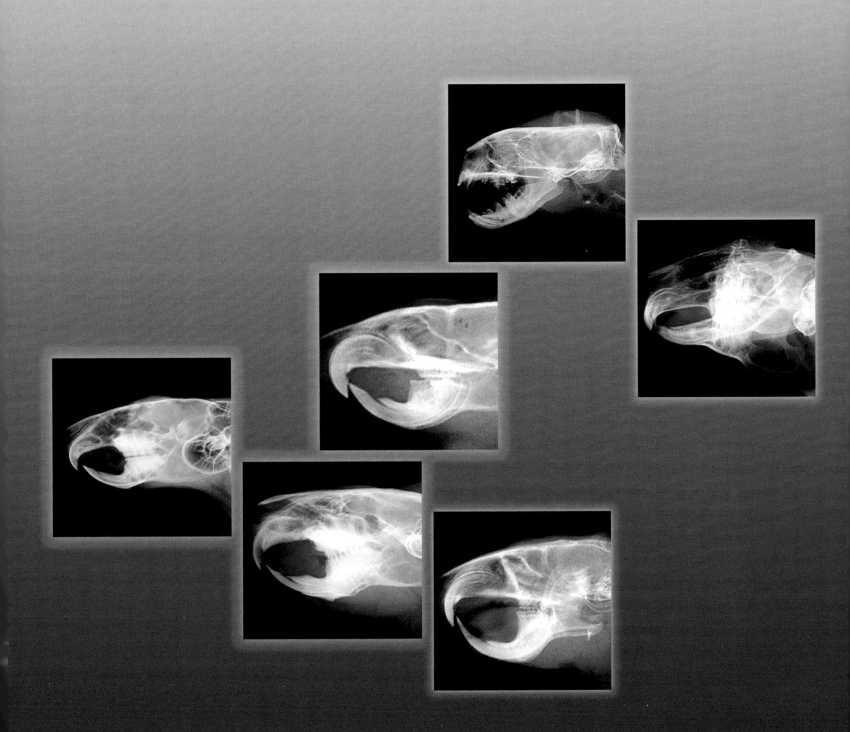

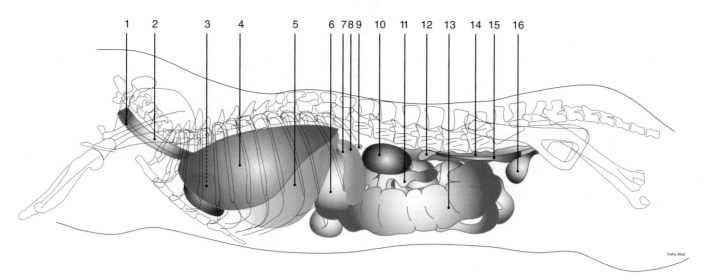

Figure 4-1, A Anatomic drawing (view of the left side) of viscera of the thorax and abdomen of an adult female hamster.

1. Trachea
2. Esophagus
3. Heart
4. Lung
5. Liver
6. Stomach
7. Pancreas
8. Spleen
9. Left adrenal gland
10. Left kidney
11. Small intestine
12. Left ovary
13. Cecum
14. Descending colon
15. Left horn of uterus
16. Urinary bladder

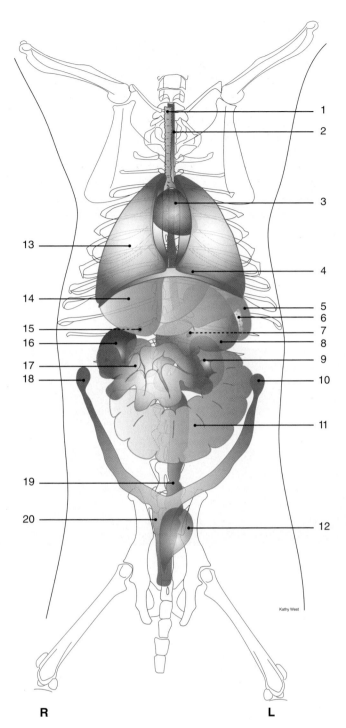

Kathy West

R   L

Figure 4-1, B Anatomic drawing (ventrodorsal view) of viscera of the thorax and abdomen of an adult female hamster.

1. Trachea
2. Esophagus
3. Heart
4. Diaphragm
5. Spleen
6. Pancreas
7. Left adrenal gland
8. Stomach
9. Left kidney
10. Left ovary
11. Cecum
12. Urinary bladder
13. Lung
14. Liver
15. Right adrenal gland
16. Right kidney
17. Small intestine
18. Right ovary
19. Descending colon
20. Body of uterus

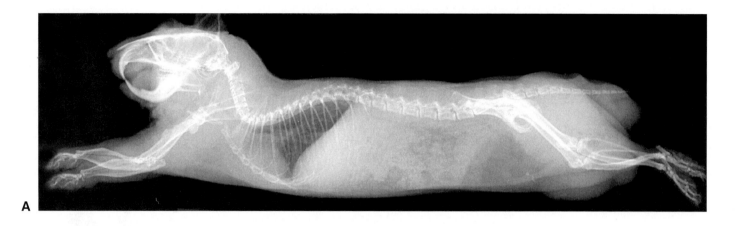

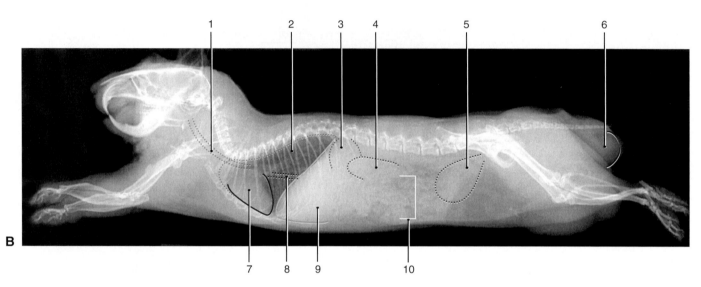

Figure 4-2, A and B
Type of animal: Hamster
Type of study: Viscera of thorax and abdomen
Projection: Laterolateral (right lateral recumbency)
Weight of animal: 150 g
Gender: Male
Reproductive status: Intact
Age: Adult

1. Trachea
2. Lung
3. Stomach
4. Kidney
5. Urinary bladder
6. Scrotum
7. Heart
8. Caudal vena cava
9. Liver
10. Cecum

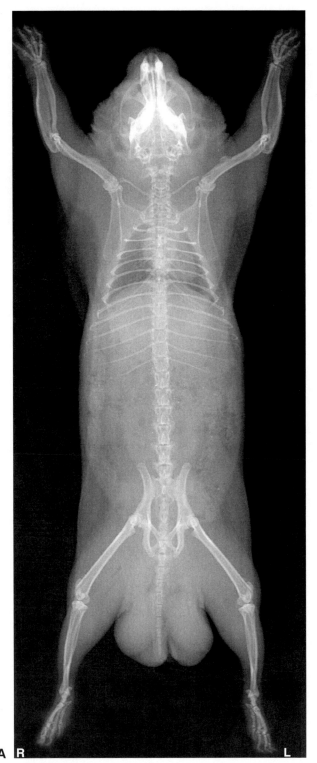

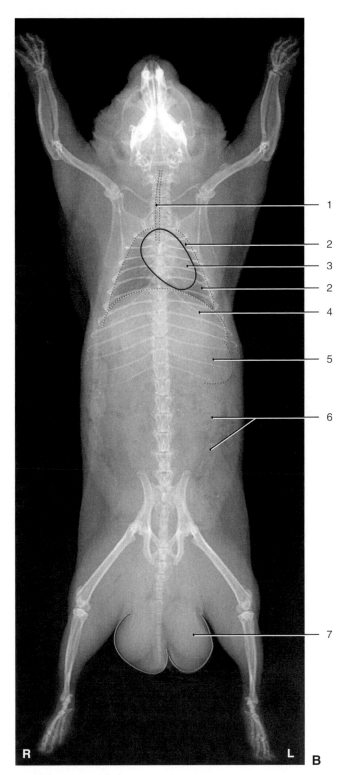

Figure 4-3, A
Type of animal: Hamster
Type of study: Viscera of thorax and abdomen
Projection: Ventrodorsal
Weight of animal: 150 g
Gender: Male
Reproductive status: Intact
Age: Adult

Figure 4-3, B
Type of animal: Hamster
Type of study: Viscera of thorax and abdomen
Projection: Ventrodorsal
Weight of animal: 150 g
Gender: Male
Reproductive status: Intact
Age: Adult

1. Trachea	5. Stomach
2. Lung	6. Cecum
3. Heart	7. Scrotum
4. Liver	

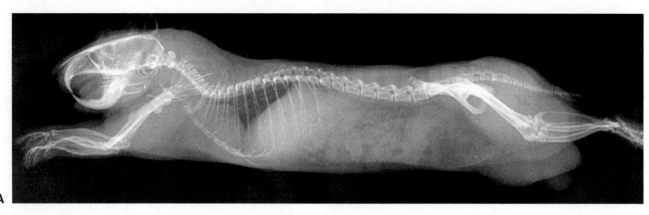

Figure 4-4, A
Type of animal: Hamster
Type of study: Whole body skeleton
Projection: Laterolateral (right lateral recumbency)
Weight of animal: 150 g
Gender: Male
Reproductive status: Intact
Age: Adult

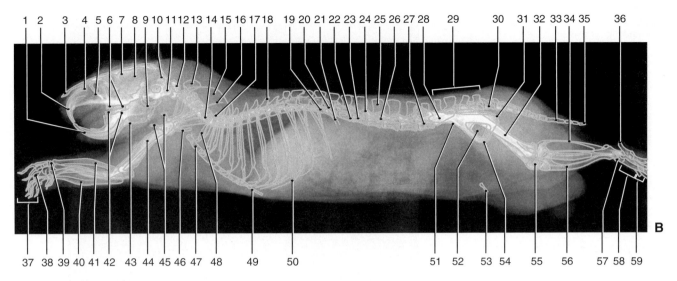

Figure 4-4, B
Type of animal: Hamster
Type of study: Whole body skeleton
Projection: Laterolateral (right lateral recumbency)
Weight of animal: 150 g
Gender: Male
Reproductive status: Intact
Age: Adult

1. Mandibular incisor tooth
2. Maxillary incisor tooth
3. Nasal bone
4. Incisive bone
5. Maxilla
6. Maxillary molar teeth
7. Frontal bone
8. Parietal bone
9. Tympanic bulla
10. Occipital bone
11. Occipital condyle
12. Dorsal tubercle of atlas
13. Spinous process of axis
14. 7th cervical vertebra
15. Scapula
16. Spine of scapula
17. 1st thoracic vertebra
18. Spinous process of thoracic vertebra
19. 13th thoracic vertebra
20. 1st lumbar vertebra

21. 13th rib
22. Lumbar intervertebral space
23. Transverse process of lumbar vertebra
24. Mammillary process of lumbar vertebra
25. Spinous process of lumbar vertebra
26. Lumbar intervertebral foramen
27. 7th lumbar vertebra
28. Sacrum
29. Spinous processes of sacral vertebrae
30. 1st caudal vertebra
31. Ischium
32. Femur
33. Caudal intervertebral space
34. Fibula
35. Caudal vertebra
36. Calcaneus
37. Phalanges
38. Metacarpal bone
39. Carpal bone
40. Ulna

41. Radius
42. Mandibular molar teeth
43. Mandible
44. Humerus
45. Clavicles
46. Suprahamate process
47. Manubrium of sternum
48. 1st rib
49. Xyphoid process
50. Costal cartilage
51. Ilium
52. Obturator foramen
53. Os penis
54. Pubis
55. Patella
56. Tibia
57. Tarsal bone
58. Metatarsal bones
59. Phalanges

Figure 4-5, A
Type of animal: Hamster
Type of study: Whole body skeleton
Projection: Ventrodorsal
Weight of animal: 150 g
Gender: Male
Reproductive status: Intact
Age: Adult

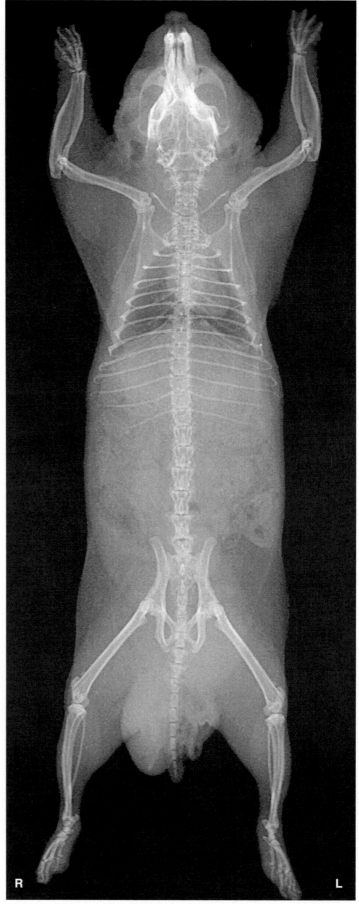

A   R   L

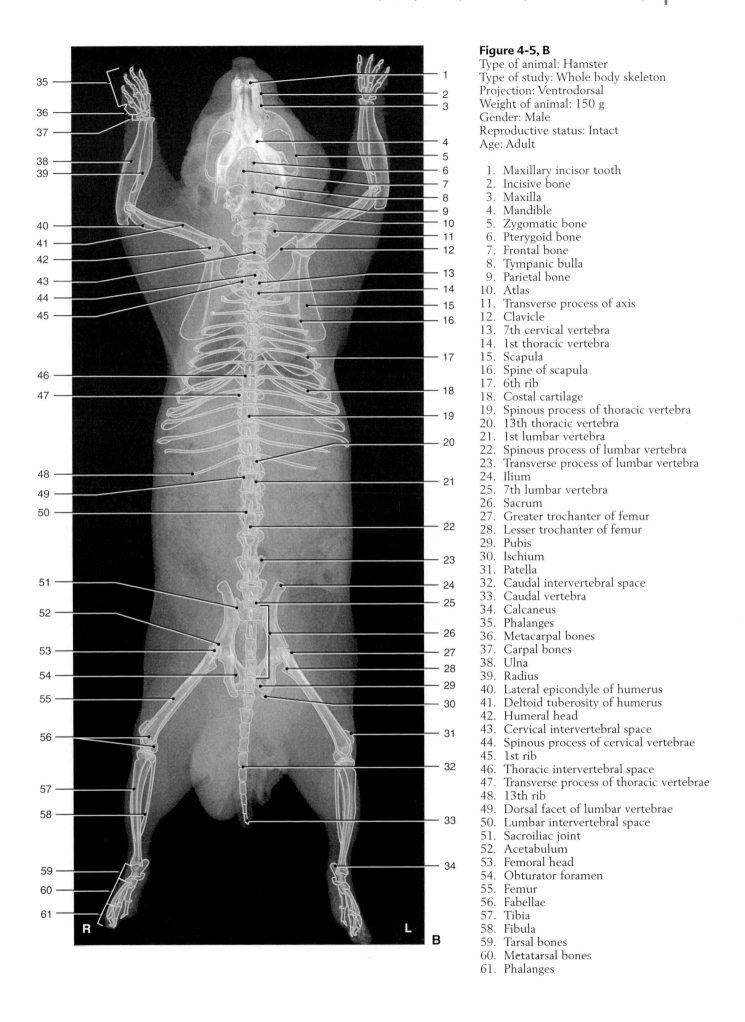

Figure 4-5, B
Type of animal: Hamster
Type of study: Whole body skeleton
Projection: Ventrodorsal
Weight of animal: 150 g
Gender: Male
Reproductive status: Intact
Age: Adult

1. Maxillary incisor tooth
2. Incisive bone
3. Maxilla
4. Mandible
5. Zygomatic bone
6. Pterygoid bone
7. Frontal bone
8. Tympanic bulla
9. Parietal bone
10. Atlas
11. Transverse process of axis
12. Clavicle
13. 7th cervical vertebra
14. 1st thoracic vertebra
15. Scapula
16. Spine of scapula
17. 6th rib
18. Costal cartilage
19. Spinous process of thoracic vertebra
20. 13th thoracic vertebra
21. 1st lumbar vertebra
22. Spinous process of lumbar vertebra
23. Transverse process of lumbar vertebra
24. Ilium
25. 7th lumbar vertebra
26. Sacrum
27. Greater trochanter of femur
28. Lesser trochanter of femur
29. Pubis
30. Ischium
31. Patella
32. Caudal intervertebral space
33. Caudal vertebra
34. Calcaneus
35. Phalanges
36. Metacarpal bones
37. Carpal bones
38. Ulna
39. Radius
40. Lateral epicondyle of humerus
41. Deltoid tuberosity of humerus
42. Humeral head
43. Cervical intervertebral space
44. Spinous process of cervical vertebrae
45. 1st rib
46. Thoracic intervertebral space
47. Transverse process of thoracic vertebrae
48. 13th rib
49. Dorsal facet of lumbar vertebrae
50. Lumbar intervertebral space
51. Sacroiliac joint
52. Acetabulum
53. Femoral head
54. Obturator foramen
55. Femur
56. Fabellae
57. Tibia
58. Fibula
59. Tarsal bones
60. Metatarsal bones
61. Phalanges

Figure 4-6, A
Type of animal: Hamster
Type of study: Head
Projection: Laterolateral
    (right lateral recumbency)
Weight of animal: 130 g
Gender: Female
Reproductive status: Intact
Age: Adult

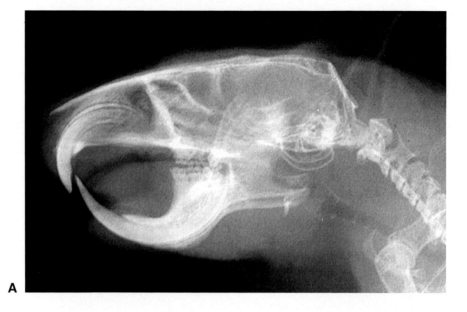

Figure 4-6, B
Type of animal: Hamster
Type of study: Head
Projection: Laterolateral
    (right lateral recumbency)
Weight of animal: 130 g
Gender: Female
Reproductive status: Intact
Age: Adult

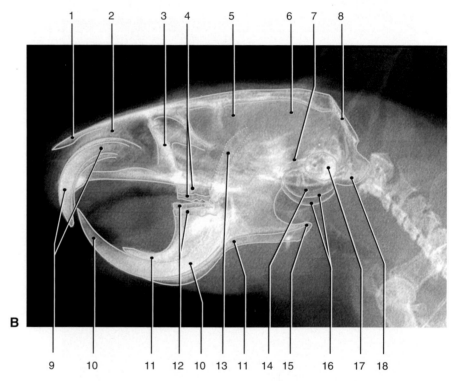

1. Nasal bone
2. Incisive bone
3. Zygomatic process of maxilla
4. Maxillary molar teeth
5. Frontal bone
6. Parietal bone
7. Temporal bone
8. Occipital bone
9. Maxillary incisor tooth
10. Mandibular incisor tooth
11. Mandible
12. Mandibular molar teeth
13. Coronoid process of mandible
14. Tympanic cavity
15. Angular process of mandible
16. Tympanic bullae
17. Petrous part of temporal bone
18. Occipital condyle

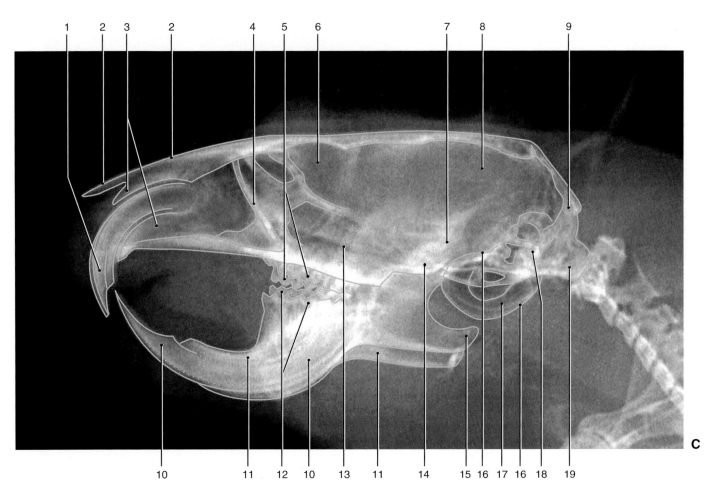

Figure 4-6, C
Type of animal: Hamster
Type of study: Magnification study of head
Projection: Laterolateral (right lateral recumbency)
Weight of animal: 130 g
Gender: Female
Reproductive status: Intact
Age: Adult

1. Maxillary incisor tooth
2. Nasal bone
3. Incisive bone
4. Zygomatic process of maxilla
5. Maxillary molar teeth
6. Frontal bone
7. Temporal bone
8. Parietal bone
9. Occipital bone
10. Mandibular incisor tooth
11. Mandible
12. Mandibular molar teeth
13. Coronoid process of mandible
14. Condylar process of mandible
15. Angular process of mandible
16. Tympanic bulla
17. Tympanic cavity
18. Petrous part of temporal bone
19. Occipital condyle

Figure 4-7, A
Type of animal: Hamster
Type of study: Head
Projection: Dorsoventral
Weight of animal: 130 g
Gender: Female
Reproductive status: Intact
Age: Adult

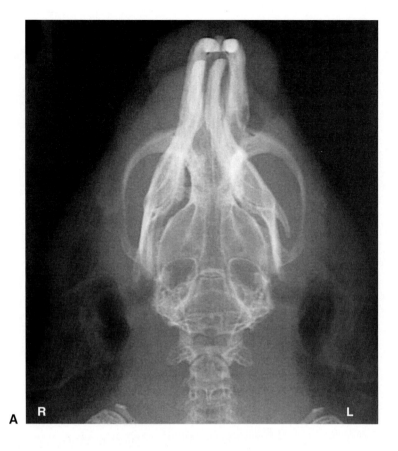

Figure 4-7, B
Type of animal: Hamster
Type of study: Head
Projection: Dorsoventral
Weight of animal: 130 g
Gender: Female
Reproductive status: Intact
Age: Adult

1. Incisive bone
2. Mandibular symphysis
3. Maxilla
4. Mandible
5. Zygomatic process of maxilla
6. Coronoid process of mandible
7. Basisphenoidal bone
8. Tympanic cavity
9. Parietal bone
10. Hyoid bones
11. Paracondylar process of
    occipital bone
12. Occipital condyle
13. Foramen magnum
14. Nasal bone
15. Maxillary incisor tooth
16. Mandibular incisor tooth
17. Nasal cavity
18. Palatine bone
19. Zygomatic bone
20. Pterygoid bone
21. Tympanic bulla
22. Angular process of mandible
23. Ear canal
24. Occipital bone

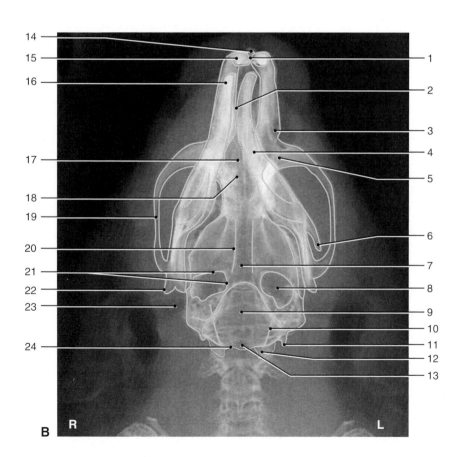

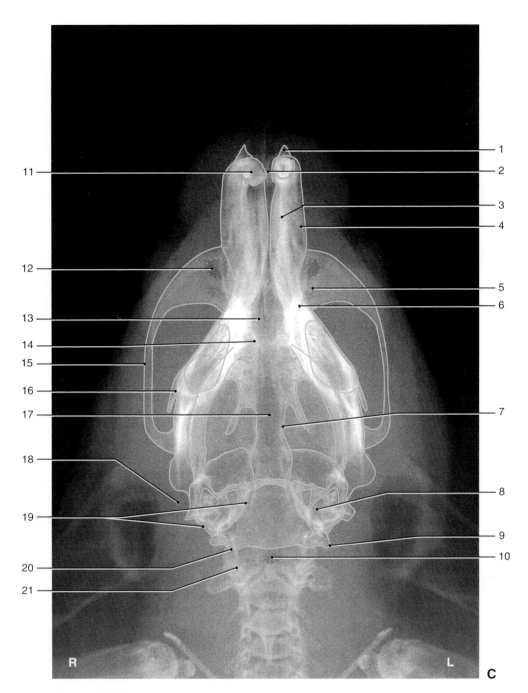

Figure 4-7, C
Type of animal: Hamster
Type of study: Magnification study of head
Projection: Dorsoventral
Weight of animal: 130 g
Gender: Female
Reproductive status: Intact
Age: Adult

1. Nasal bone
2. Incisive bone
3. Mandibular incisor tooth
4. Maxilla
5. Zygomatic process of maxilla
6. Mandible
7. Pterygoid bone
8. Petrous part of temporal bone
9. Paracondylar process of occipital bone
10. Foramen magnum
11. Maxillary incisor tooth
12. Infraorbital hiatus
13. Nasal cavity
14. Palatine bone
15. Zygomatic bone
16. Coronoid process of mandible
17. Basisphenoidal bone
18. Ear canal
19. Tympanic bulla
20. Occipital bone
21. Occipital condyle

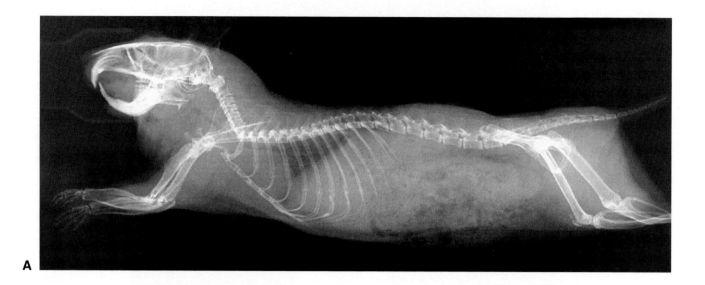

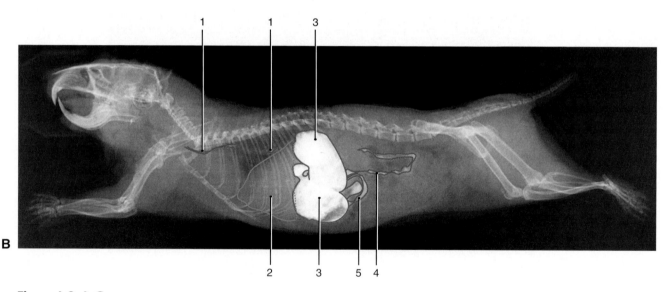

Figure 4-8, A-G
Type of animal: Hamster
Type of study: Gastrointestinal positive contrast study
Contrast medium: Barium sulfate suspension (Novopaque
  60% w/v; Lafayette Pharmaceutical, Inc., Lafayette, Ind.)
  4 ml administered via esophageal gavage
Projection: Laterolateral (right lateral recumbency)
Weight of animal: 190 g
Gender: Female
Reproductive status: Intact
Age: 1.3 years

1. Esophagus
2. Liver
3. Stomach
4. Duodenum
5. Small intestine
6. Cecum
7. Colon
8. Rectum

Image	Time (hr)
A	Survey
B	0.25

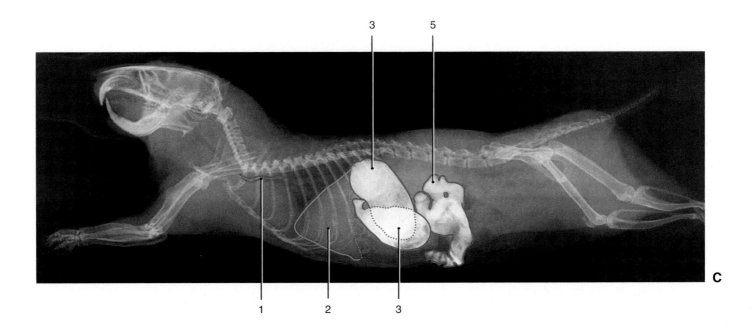

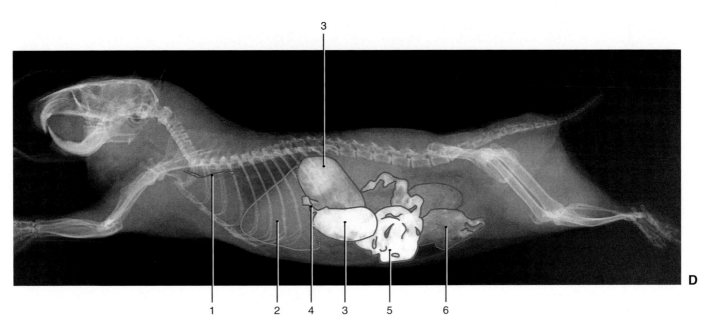

Figure 4-8, A-G—cont'd

Type of animal: Hamster
Type of study: Gastrointestinal positive contrast study
Contrast medium: Barium sulfate suspension (Novopaque
   60% w/v; Lafayette Pharmaceutical, Inc., Lafayette, Ind.)
   4 ml administered via esophageal gavage
Projection: Laterolateral (right lateral recumbency)
Weight of animal: 190 g
Gender: Female
Reproductive status: Intact
Age: 1.3 years

1. Esophagus
2. Liver
3. Stomach
4. Duodenum
5. Small intestine
6. Cecum
7. Colon
8. Rectum

Image	Time (hr)
C	0.67
D	1.75

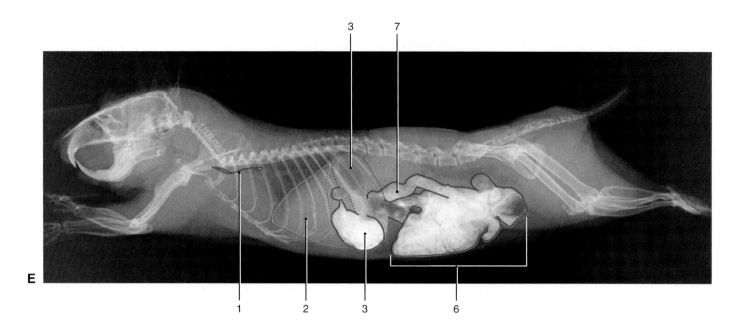

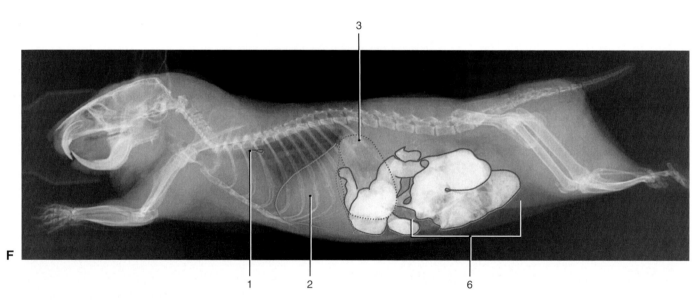

Figure 4-8, A-G—cont'd

Type of animal: Hamster
Type of study: Gastrointestinal positive contrast study
Contrast medium: Barium sulfate suspension (Novopaque 60% w/v; Lafayette Pharmaceutical, Inc., Lafayette, Ind.) 4 ml administered via esophageal gavage
Projection: Laterolateral (right lateral recumbency)
Weight of animal: 190 g
Gender: Female
Reproductive status: Intact
Age: 1.3 years

1. Esophagus
2. Liver
3. Stomach
4. Duodenum
5. Small intestine
6. Cecum
7. Colon
8. Rectum

Image	Time (hr)
E	3.25
F	4.25

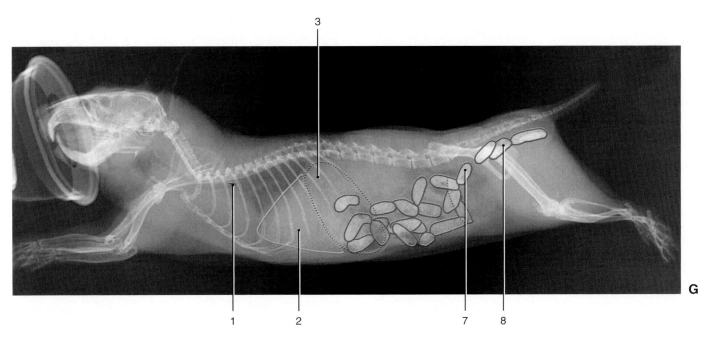

Figure 4-8, A-G—cont'd
Type of animal: Hamster
Type of study: Gastrointestinal positive contrast study
Contrast medium: Barium sulfate suspension (Novopaque
  60% w/v; Lafayette Pharmaceutical, Inc., Lafayette, Ind.)
  4 ml administered via esophageal gavage
Projection: Laterolateral (right lateral recumbency)
Weight of animal: 190 g
Gender: Female
Reproductive status: Intact
Age: 1.3 years

1. Esophagus
2. Liver
3. Stomach
4. Duodenum
5. Small intestine
6. Cecum
7. Colon
8. Rectum

Image	Time (hr)
G	23.00

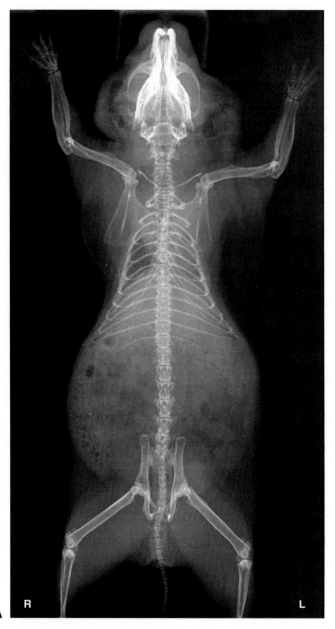

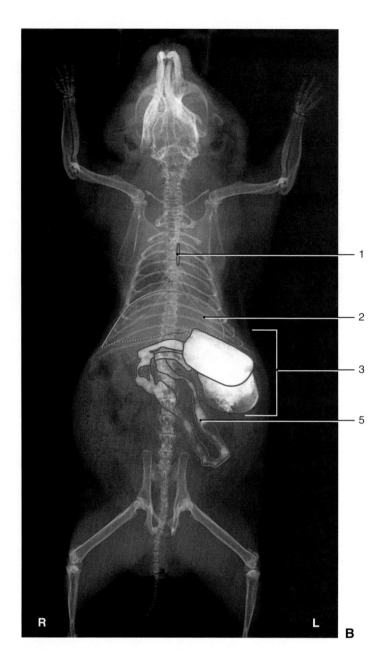

Figure 4-9, A-G
Type of animal: Hamster
Type of study: Gastrointestinal positive contrast study
Contrast medium: Barium sulfate suspension (Novopaque
    60% w/v; Lafayette Pharmaceutical, Inc., Lafayette, Ind.)
    4 ml administered via esophageal gavage
Projection: Ventrodorsal
Weight of animal: 190 g
Gender: Female
Reproductive status: Intact
Age: 1.3 years

1. Esophagus
2. Liver
3. Stomach
4. Duodenum
5. Small intestine
6. Cecum
7. Colon
8. Rectum

Image	Time (hr)
A	Survey
B	0.25

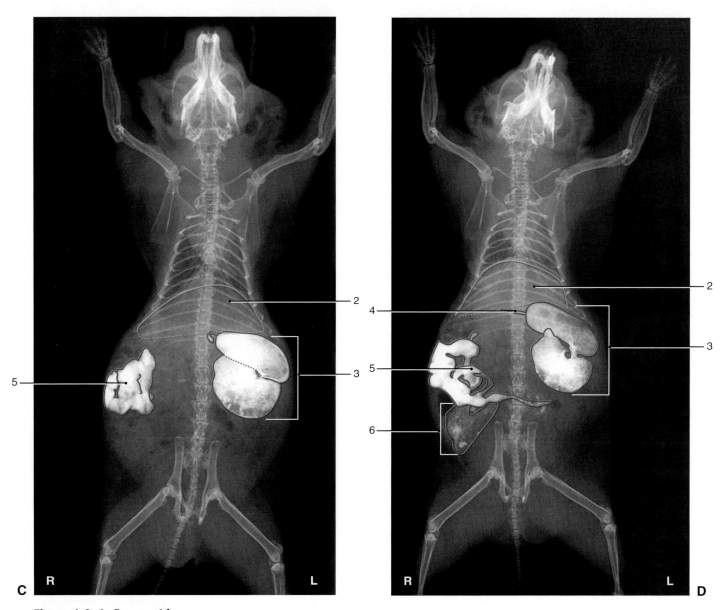

Figure 4-9, A-G—cont'd
Type of animal: Hamster
Type of study: Gastrointestinal positive contrast study
Contrast medium: Barium sulfate suspension (Novopaque
    60% w/v; Lafayette Pharmaceutical, Inc., Lafayette, Ind.)
    4 ml administered via esophageal gavage
Projection: Ventrodorsal
Weight of animal: 190 g
Gender: Female
Reproductive status: Intact
Age: 1.3 years

1. Esophagus
2. Liver
3. Stomach
4. Duodenum
5. Small intestine
6. Cecum
7. Colon
8. Rectum

Image	Time (hr)
C	0.67
D	1.75

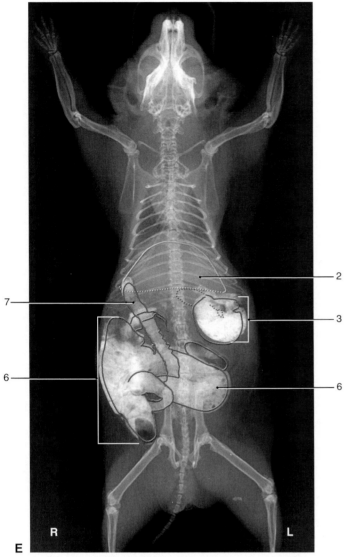

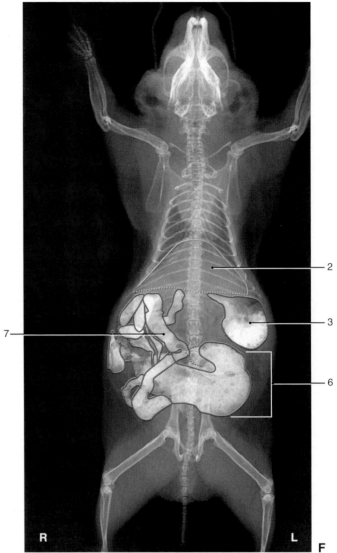

Figure 4-9, A-G—cont'd

Type of animal: Hamster
Type of study: Gastrointestinal positive contrast study
Contrast medium: Barium sulfate suspension (Novopaque
   60% w/v; Lafayette Pharmaceutical, Inc., Lafayette, Ind.)
   4 ml administered via esophageal gavage
Projection: Ventrodorsal
Weight of animal: 190 g
Gender: Female
Reproductive status: Intact
Age: 1.3 years

1. Esophagus
2. Liver
3. Stomach
4. Duodenum
5. Small intestine
6. Cecum
7. Colon
8. Rectum

Image	Time (hr)
E	3.25
F	4.25

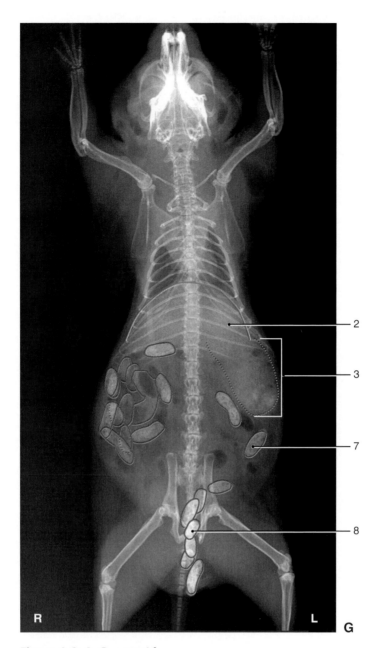

Figure 4-9, A-G—cont'd
Type of animal: Hamster
Type of study: Gastrointestinal positive contrast study
Contrast medium: Barium sulfate suspension (Novopaque
    60% w/v; Lafayette Pharmaceutical, Inc., Lafayette, Ind.)
    4 ml administered via esophageal gavage
Projection: Ventrodorsal
Weight of animal: 190 g
Gender: Female
Reproductive status: Intact
Age: 1.3 years

Image	Time (hr)
G	23.00

1. Esophagus
2. Liver
3. Stomach
4. Duodenum
5. Small intestine
6. Cecum
7. Colon
8. Rectum

CHAPTER 5

Domestic Chinchilla *(Chinchilla lanigera)*

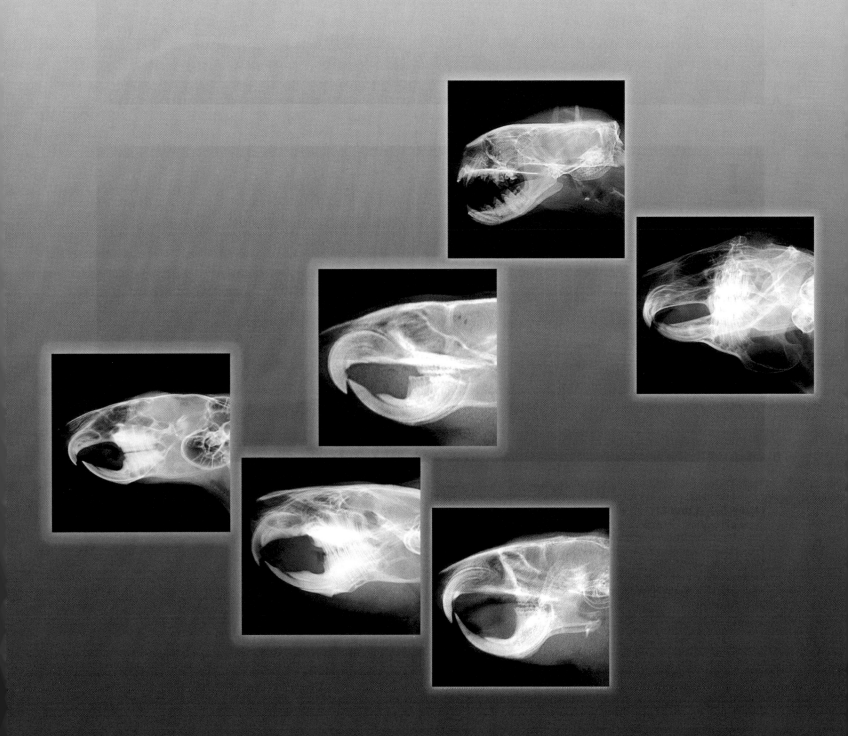

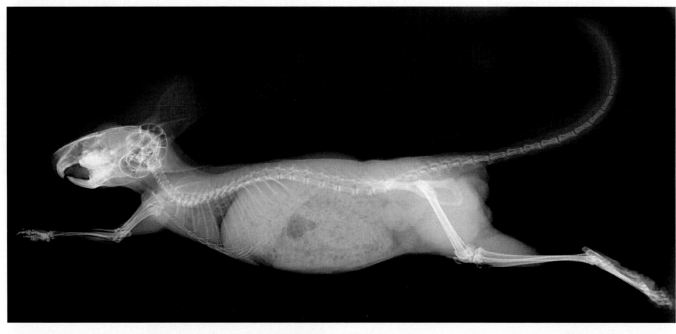

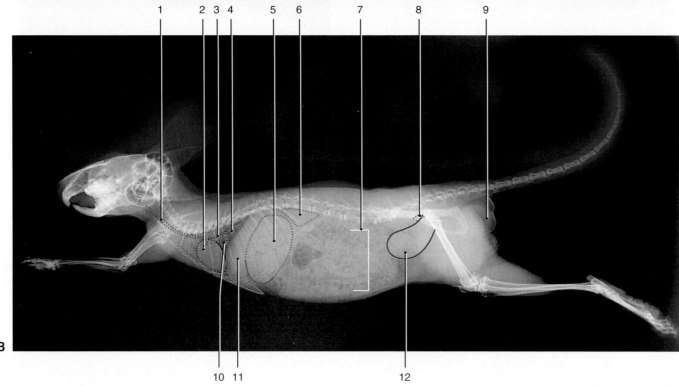

Figure 5-1, A and B

Type of animal: Chinchilla
Type of study: Viscera of thorax and abdomen
Projection: Laterolateral (right lateral recumbency)
Weight of animal: 486 g
Gender: Male
Reproductive status: Neutered
Age: Adult

1. Trachea
2. Heart
3. Pulmonary vein
4. Lung
5. Stomach
6. Spleen
7. Cecum
8. Colon
9. Scrotum
10. Caudal vena cava
11. Liver
12. Urinary bladder

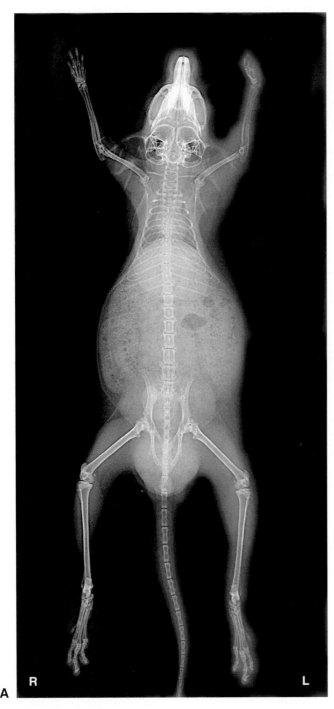

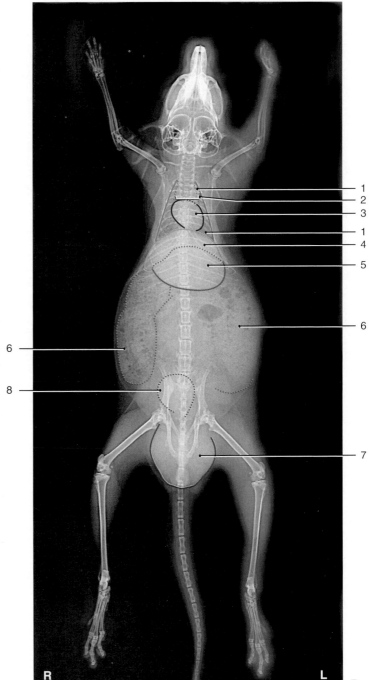

Figure 5-2, A
Type of animal: Chinchilla
Type of study: Viscera of thorax and abdomen
Projection: Ventrodorsal
Weight of animal: 486 g
Gender: Male
Reproductive status: Intact
Age: Adult

Figure 5-2, B
Type of animal: Chinchilla
Type of study: Viscera of thorax and abdomen
Projection: Ventrodorsal
Weight of animal: 486 g
Gender: Male
Reproductive status: Intact
Age: Adult

1. Lung
2. Cranial mediastinum
3. Heart
4. Liver
5. Stomach
6. Cecum
7. Scrotum
8. Urinary bladder

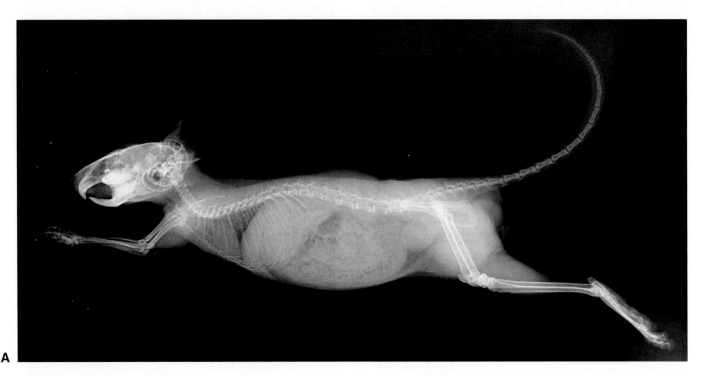

Figure 5-3, A
Type of animal: Chinchilla
Type of study: Whole body skeleton
Projection: Laterolateral (right lateral recumbency)
Weight of animal: 486 g
Gender: Male
Reproductive status: Intact
Age: Adult

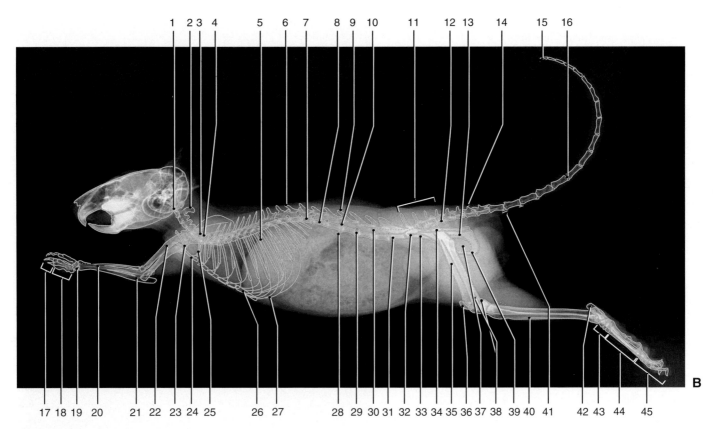

Figure 5-3, B
Type of animal: Chinchilla
Type of study: Whole body skeleton
Projection: Laterolateral (right lateral recumbency)
Weight of animal: 486 g
Gender: Male
Reproductive status: Intact
Age: Adult

1. Atlas
2. Spinous process of axis
3. 7th cervical vertebra
4. 1st thoracic vertebra
5. Rib
6. Spinous process of thoracic vertebra
7. 14th thoracic vertebra
8. 1st lumbar vertebra
9. Spinous process of lumbar vertebra
10. Lumbar intervertebral foramen
11. Spinous processes of sacral vertebrae
12. 1st caudal vertebra
13. Ischium
14. Articular process of caudal vertebra
15. Caudal vertebra
16. Caudal intervertebral space
17. Phalanges
18. Metacarpal bones
19. Carpal bones
20. Radius
21. Ulna
22. Humerus
23. Clavicle
24. Manubrium of sternum
25. 1st rib
26. Xyphoid process
27. Costal cartilage
28. Transverse process of lumbar vertebra
29. Lumbar intervertebral space
30. Spinal canal
31. 6th lumbar vertebra
32. Sacrum
33. Ilium
34. Greater trochanter of femur
35. Femur
36. Patella
37. Obturator foramen
38. Fabellae
39. Pubis
40. Tibia
41. Transverse process of caudal vertebra
42. Calcaneus
43. Tarsal bones
44. Metatarsal bones
45. Phalanges

Figure 5-4, A
Type of animal: Chinchilla
Type of study: Whole body skeleton
Projection: Ventrodorsal
Weight of animal: 486 g
Gender: Male
Reproductive status: Intact
Age: Adult

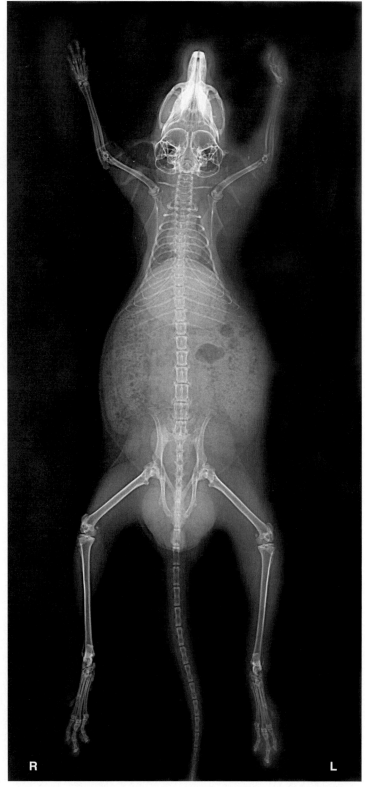

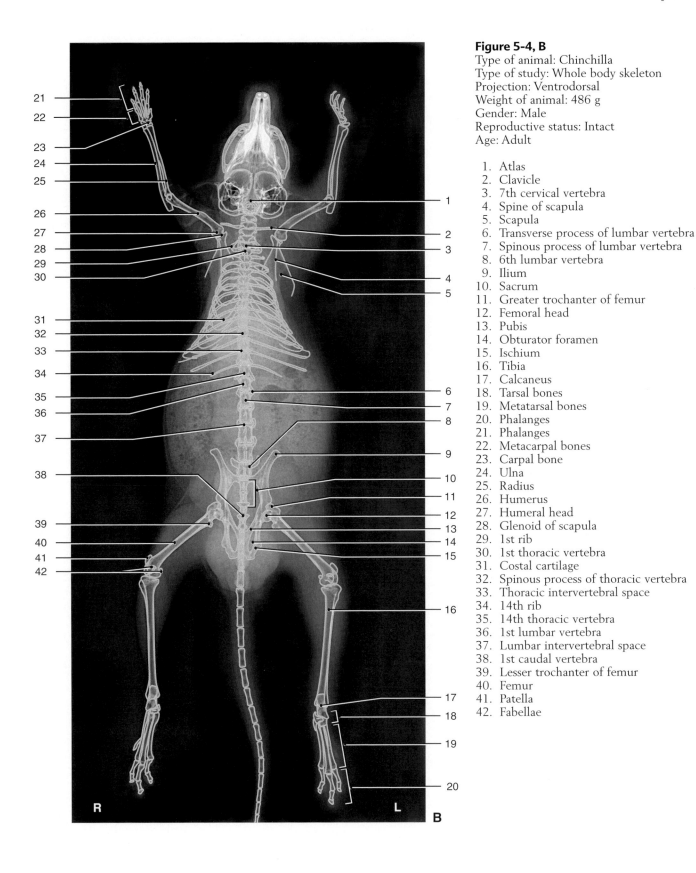

Figure 5-4, B
Type of animal: Chinchilla
Type of study: Whole body skeleton
Projection: Ventrodorsal
Weight of animal: 486 g
Gender: Male
Reproductive status: Intact
Age: Adult

1. Atlas
2. Clavicle
3. 7th cervical vertebra
4. Spine of scapula
5. Scapula
6. Transverse process of lumbar vertebra
7. Spinous process of lumbar vertebra
8. 6th lumbar vertebra
9. Ilium
10. Sacrum
11. Greater trochanter of femur
12. Femoral head
13. Pubis
14. Obturator foramen
15. Ischium
16. Tibia
17. Calcaneus
18. Tarsal bones
19. Metatarsal bones
20. Phalanges
21. Phalanges
22. Metacarpal bones
23. Carpal bone
24. Ulna
25. Radius
26. Humerus
27. Humeral head
28. Glenoid of scapula
29. 1st rib
30. 1st thoracic vertebra
31. Costal cartilage
32. Spinous process of thoracic vertebra
33. Thoracic intervertebral space
34. 14th rib
35. 14th thoracic vertebra
36. 1st lumbar vertebra
37. Lumbar intervertebral space
38. 1st caudal vertebra
39. Lesser trochanter of femur
40. Femur
41. Patella
42. Fabellae

Figure 5-5, A
Type of animal: Chinchilla
Type of study: Head
Projection: Laterolateral
   (right lateral recumbency)
Weight of animal: 486 g
Gender: Male
Reproductive status: Intact
Age: Adult

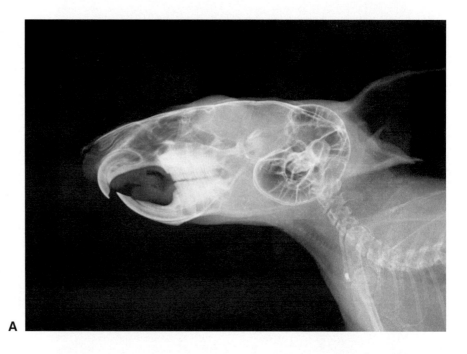

Figure 5-5, B
Type of animal: Chinchilla
Type of study: Head
Projection: Laterolateral
   (right lateral recumbency)
Weight of animal: 486 g
Gender: Male
Reproductive status: Intact
Age: Adult

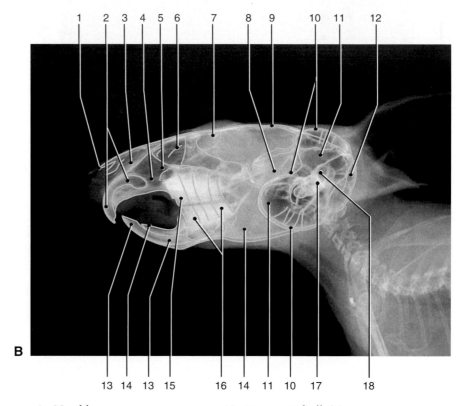

1. Nasal bone	10. Tympanic bulla(e)
2. Maxillary incisor tooth	11. Tympanic cavity
3. Incisive bone	12. Occipital bone
4. Maxilla	13. Mandibular incisor tooth
5. Nasal cavity	14. Mandible
6. Ethmoturbinates	15. Maxillary premolar tooth
7. Frontal bone	16. Mandibular premolar and molar teeth
8. Temporal bone	17. Petrous part of temporal bone
9. Parietal bone	18. External acoustic meatus

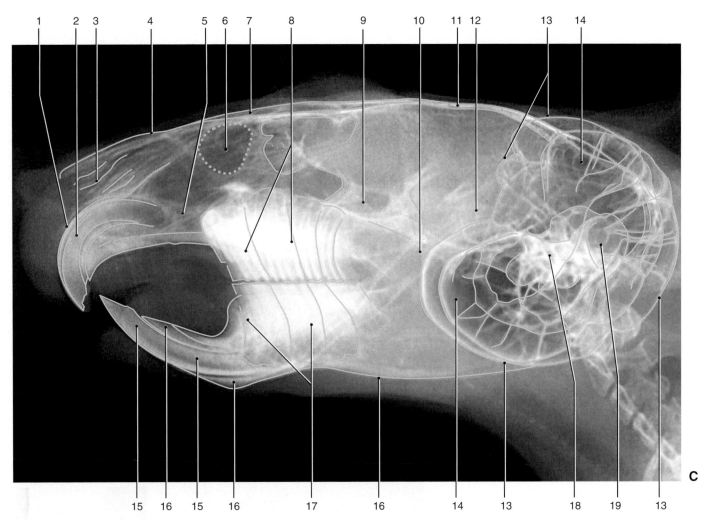

Figure 5-5, C
Type of animal: Chinchilla
Type of study: Magnification study of head
Projection: Laterolateral (right lateral recumbency)
Weight of animal: 430 g
Gender: Male
Reproductive status: Intact
Age: Juvenile

1. Incisive bone
2. Maxillary incisor tooth
3. Nasoturbinates
4. Nasal bone
5. Maxilla
6. Infraorbital hiatus
7. Frontal bone
8. Maxillary premolar and molar teeth
9. Zygomatic bone
10. Coronoid process of mandible
11. Parietal bone
12. Temporal bone
13. Tympanic bulla(e)
14. Tympanic cavity
15. Mandibular incisor tooth
16. Mandible
17. Mandibular premolar and molar teeth
18. Petrous part of temporal bone
19. External acoustic meatus

Figure 5-6, A
Type of animal: Chinchilla
Type of study: Head
Projection: Oblique
(30 degree) ventrodorsal
Weight of animal: 486 g
Gender: Male
Reproductive status: Intact
Age: Adult

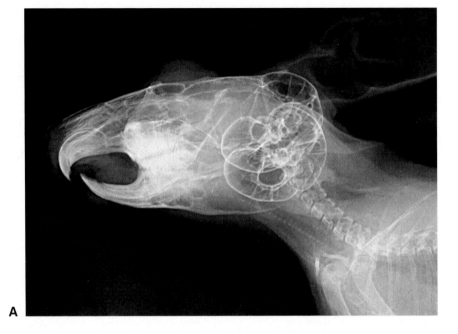

A

Figure 5-6, B
Type of animal: Chinchilla
Type of study: Head
Projection: Oblique
(30 degree) ventrodorsal
Weight of animal: 486 g
Gender: Male
Reproductive status: Intact
Age: Adult

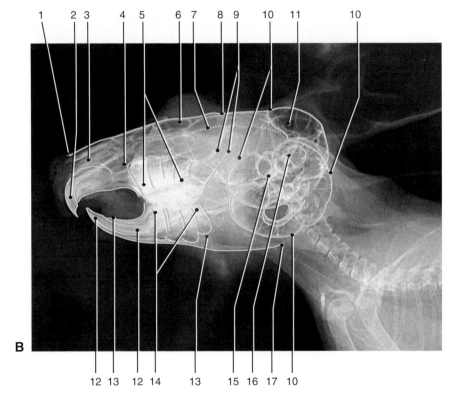

B

1. Nasal bone
2. Maxillary incisor tooth
3. Incisive bone
4. Maxilla
5. Maxillary premolar and molar teeth
6. Frontal bone
7. Zygomatic bone
8. Parietal bone
9. Coronoid processes of mandible
10. Tympanic bulla
11. Tympanic cavity
12. Mandibular incisor tooth
13. Mandible
14. Mandibular premolar and molar teeth
15. Petrous part of temporal bone
16. External acoustic meatus
17. Angular process of mandible

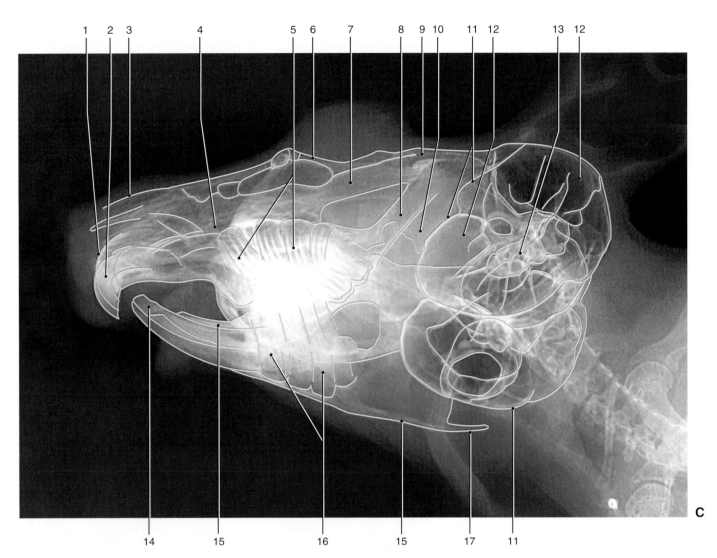

Figure 5-6, C
Type of animal: Chinchilla
Type of study: Magnification study of head
Projection: Oblique (30 degree) ventrodorsal
Weight of animal: 430 g
Gender: Male
Reproductive status: Intact
Age: Juvenile

1. Incisive bone
2. Maxillary incisor tooth
3. Nasal bone
4. Maxilla
5. Maxillary premolar and molar teeth
6. Frontal bone
7. Zygomatic bone
8. Coronoid process of mandible
9. Parietal bone
10. Temporal bone
11. Tympanic bulla
12. Tympanic cavity
13. Petrous part of temporal bone
14. Mandibular incisor tooth
15. Mandible
16. Mandibular premolar and molar teeth
17. Angular process of mandible

Figure 5-7, A
Type of animal: Chinchilla
Type of study: Head
Projection: Dorsoventral
Weight of animal: 486 g
Gender: Male
Reproductive status: Intact
Age: Adult

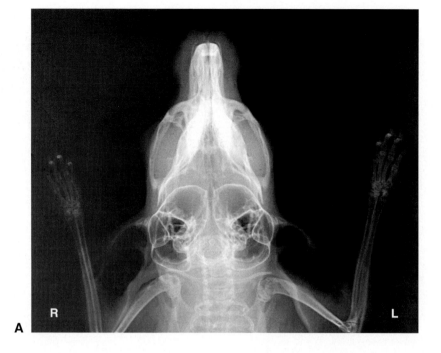

Figure 5-7, B
Type of animal: Chinchilla
Type of study: Head
Projection: Dorsoventral
Weight of animal: 486 g
Gender: Male
Reproductive status: Intact
Age: Adult

1. Maxillary incisor tooth
2. Incisive bone
3. Zygomatic process of maxilla
4. Premolar and molar teeth
5. Mandible
6. Zygomatic bone
7. Coronoid process of mandible
8. Basisphenoidal bone
9. Tympanic bulla
10. Tympanic cavity
11. Petrous part of temporal bone
12. Foramen magnum
13. Occipital bone
14. Maxilla
15. Infraorbital hiatus
16. Vomer
17. Pterygoid bone
18. Angular process of mandible
19. Ear canal

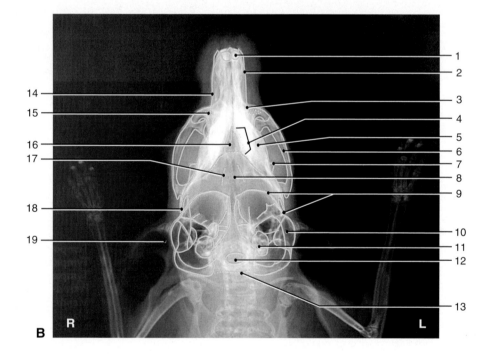

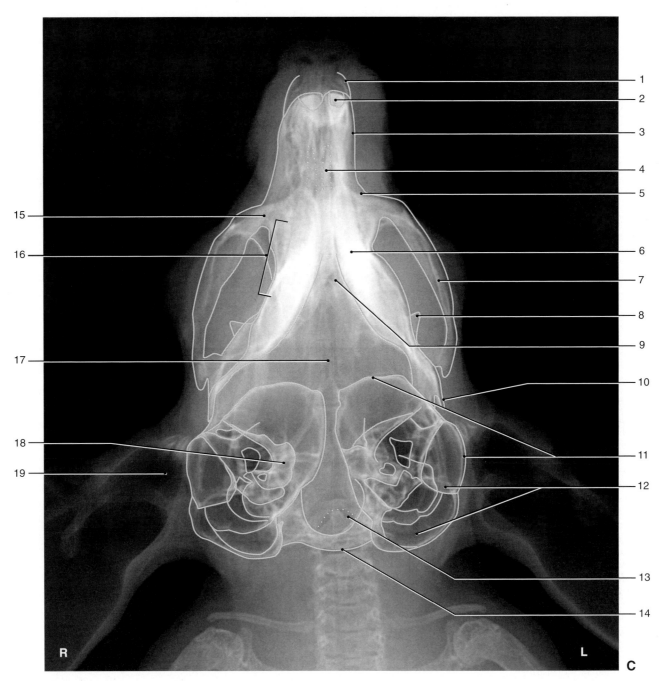

Figure 5-7, C
Type of animal: Chinchilla
Type of study: Magnification study of head
Projection: Dorsoventral
Weight of animal: 430 g
Gender: Male
Reproductive status: Intact
Age: Juvenile

1. Nasal bone
2. Maxillary incisor tooth
3. Incisive bone
4. Mandibular incisor tooth
5. Maxilla
6. Mandible
7. Zygomatic bone
8. Coronoid process of mandible
9. Palatine bone
10. Angular process of mandible
11. Tympanic bulla
12. Tympanic cavity
13. Foramen magnum
14. Occipital bone
15. Zygomatic process of maxilla
16. Premolar and molar teeth
17. Basisphenoidal bone
18. Petrous part of temporal bone
19. Ear canal

Figure 5-8, A
Type of animal: Chinchilla
Type of study: Thoracic limb
Projection: Mediolateral
Weight of animal: 486 g
Gender: Male
Reproductive status: Intact
Age: Adult

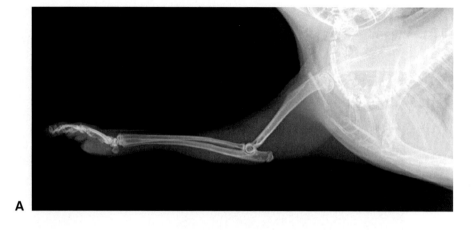

A

Figure 5-8, B
Type of animal: Chinchilla
Type of study: Thoracic limb
Projection: Mediolateral
Weight of animal: 486 g
Gender: Male
Reproductive status: Intact
Age: Adult

1. Phalanges
2. Metacarpal bones
3. Carpal bones
4. Radius
5. Humeral condyle
6. Humerus
7. Deltoid tuberosity of humerus
8. Clavicle
9. Scapula
10. Spine of scapula
11. Distal phalanx
12. Middle phalanx
13. Proximal phalanx
14. Accessory carpal bone
15. Ulna
16. Trochlear notch of ulna
17. Olecranon of ulna
18. Humeral head
19. Scapulohumeral joint space

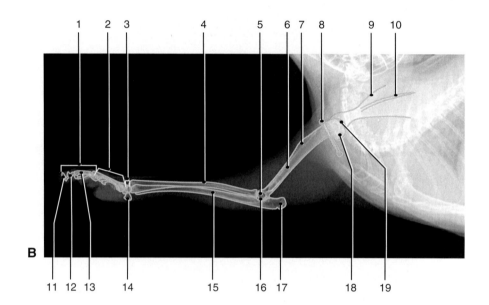

B

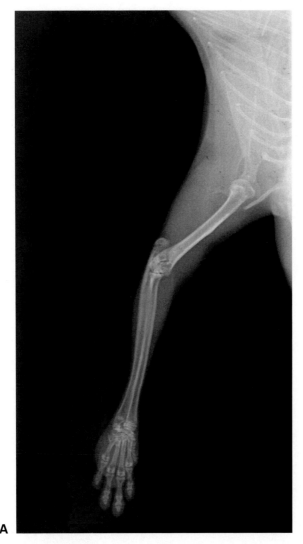

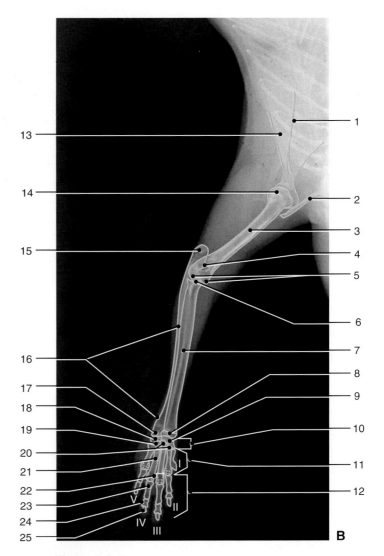

Figure 5-9, A
Type of animal: Chinchilla
Type of study: Thoracic limb
Projection: Ventrodorsal
Weight of animal: 486 g
Gender: Male
Reproductive status: Intact
Age: Adult

Figure 5-9, B
Type of animal: Chinchilla
Type of study: Thoracic limb
Projection: Ventrodorsal
Weight of animal: 486 g
Gender: Male
Reproductive status: Intact
Age: Adult

1. Spine of scapula
2. Clavicle
3. Humerus
4. Anconeal process
   of olecranon
5. Humeral condyles
6. Humeroradial joint
   space
7. Radius
8. Distal radial epiphysis
9. Intermedioradial
   carpal bone
10. Carpal bones
11. Metacarpal bones
12. Phalanges
13. Scapula
14. Humeral head
15. Olecranon of ulna
16. Ulna
17. Styloid process of ulna
18. Ulnar carpal bone
19. Carpal bone IV
20. Carpal bones I, II, and III
21. Metacarpal bone IV
22. Proximal sesamoid bones
23. Proximal phalanx of digit IV
24. Middle phalanx of digit IV
25. Distal phalanx of digit IV

Figure 5-10, A
Type of animal: Chinchilla
Type of study: Elbow joint
Projection: Mediolateral
Weight of animal: 486 g
Gender: Male
Reproductive status: Intact
Age: Adult

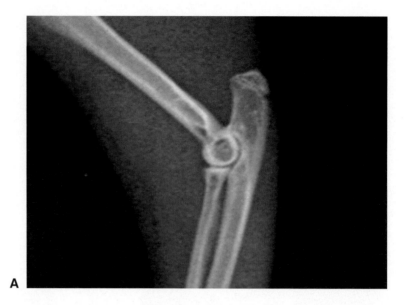

Figure 5-10, B
Type of animal: Chinchilla
Type of study: Elbow joint
Projection: Mediolateral
Weight of animal: 486 g
Gender: Male
Reproductive status: Intact
Age: Adult

1. Olecranon of ulna
2. Trochlear notch of ulna
3. Ulna
4. Humerus
5. Humeral condyle
6. Radius

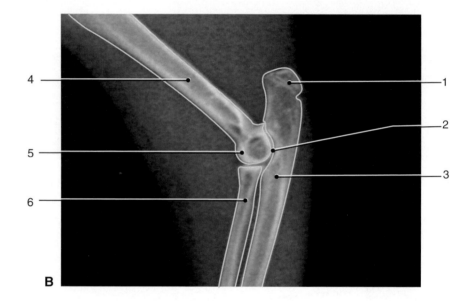

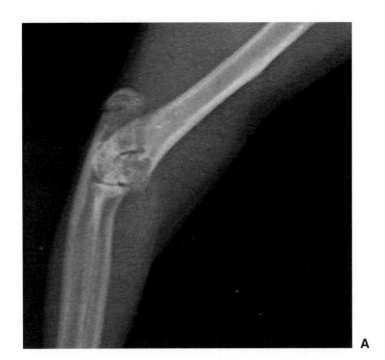

Figure 5-11, A
Type of animal: Chinchilla
Type of study: Elbow joint
Projection: Caudocranial
Weight of animal: 486 g
Gender: Male
Reproductive status: Intact
Age: Adult

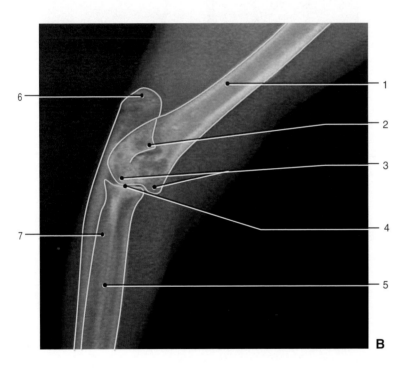

Figure 5-11, B
Type of animal: Chinchilla
Type of study: Elbow joint
Projection: Caudocranial
Weight of animal: 486 g
Gender: Male
Reproductive status: Intact
Age: Adult

1. Humerus
2. Anconeal process of olecranon
3. Humeral condyles
4. Humeroradial joint space
5. Radius
6. Olecranon of ulna
7. Ulna

Figure 5-12, A
Type of animal: Chinchilla
Type of study: Distal thoracic limb
Projection: Mediolateral
Weight of animal: 486 g
Gender: Male
Reproductive status: Intact
Age: Adult

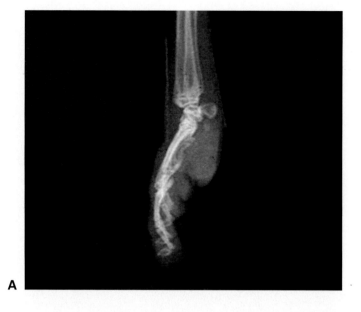

A

Figure 5-12, B
Type of animal: Chinchilla
Type of study: Distal thoracic limb
Projection: Mediolateral
Weight of animal: 486 g
Gender: Male
Reproductive status: Intact
Age: Adult

1. Ulna
2. Accessory carpal bone
3. Proximal phalanx
4. Middle phalanx
5. Distal phalanx
6. Radius
7. Carpal bones
8. Metacarpal bones
9. Phalanges

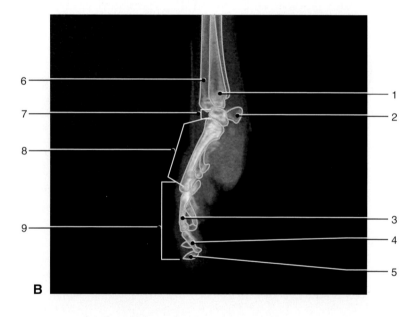

B

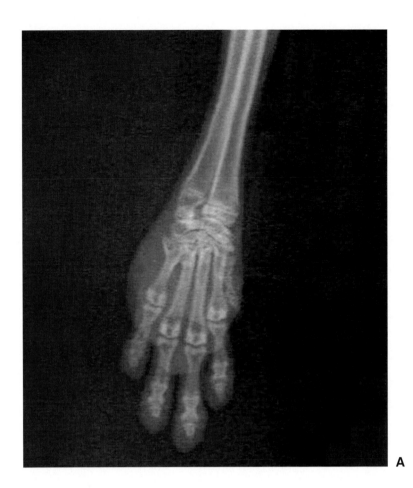

Figure 5-13, A
Type of animal: Chinchilla
Type of study: Distal thoracic limb
Projection: Dorsopalmar
Weight of animal: 486 g
Gender: Male
Reproductive status: Intact
Age: Adult

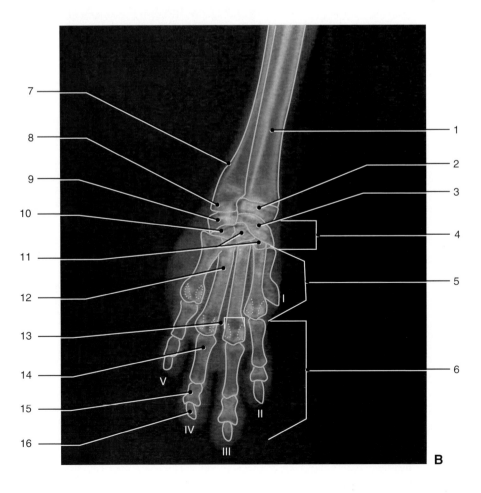

Figure 5-13, B
Type of animal: Chinchilla
Type of study: Distal thoracic limb
Projection: Dorsopalmar
Weight of animal: 486 g
Gender: Male
Reproductive status: Intact
Age: Adult

1. Radius
2. Distal radial epiphysis
3. Intermedioradial carpal bone
4. Carpal bones
5. Metacarpal bones
6. Phalanges
7. Ulna
8. Styloid process of ulna
9. Ulnar carpal bone
10. Carpal bone IV
11. Carpal bones I, II, and III
12. Metacarpal bone IV
13. Proximal sesamoid bones
14. Proximal phalanx of digit IV
15. Middle phalanx of digit IV
16. Distal phalanx of digit IV

Figure 5-14, A
Type of animal: Chinchilla
Type of study: Pelvic limb
Projection: Mediolateral
Weight of animal: 486 g
Gender: Male
Reproductive status: Intact
Age: Adult

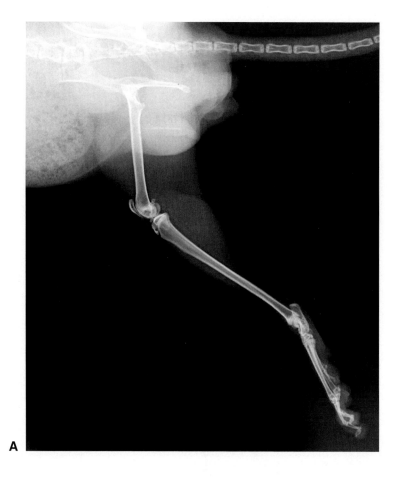

A

Figure 5-14, B
Type of animal: Chinchilla
Type of study: Pelvic limb
Projection: Mediolateral
Weight of animal: 486 g
Gender: Male
Reproductive status: Intact
Age: Adult

1. Greater trochanter of femur
2. Lesser trochanter of femur
3. Os penis
4. Femur
5. Fabella
6. Fibula
7. Calcaneal tuber
8. Talus
9. Calcaneus
10. Medial tibial bone
11. Central tarsal bone
12. Tarsal bones I, II, III, and IV
13. Digit V
14. Proximal sesamoid bone
15. Metatarsal bone
16. Proximal phalanx
17. Middle phalanx
18. Distal phalanx
19. Femoral head
20. Femoral condyles
21. Patella
22. Tibia
23. Trochlea of talus
24. Tarsal bones
25. Metatarsal bones
26. Phalanges

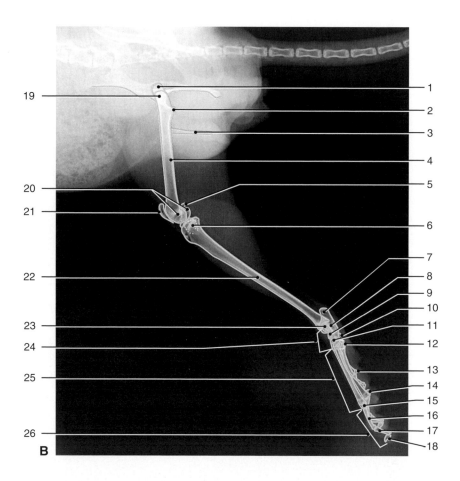

B

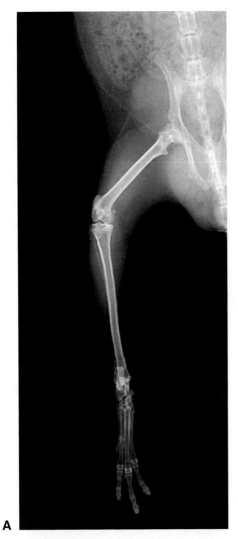

A

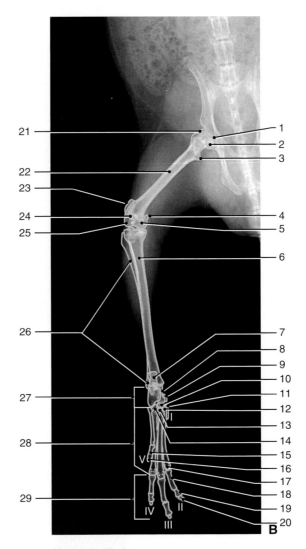

B

Figure 5-15, A
Type of animal: Chinchilla
Type of study: Pelvic limb
Projection: Ventrodorsal
Weight of animal: 486 g
Gender: Male
Reproductive status: Intact
Age: Adult

Figure 5-15, B
Type of animal: Chinchilla
Type of study: Pelvic limb
Projection: Ventrodorsal
Weight of animal: 486 g
Gender: Male
Reproductive status: Intact
Age: Adult

1. Acetabulum
2. Femoral head
3. Lesser trochanter of femur
4. Medial fabella
5. Medial femoral condyle
6. Tibia
7. Calcaneus
8. Talus
9. Medial tibial bone
10. Central tarsal bone
11. Tarsal bone I
12. Tarsal bone II
13. Tarsal bone III
14. Tarsal bone IV
15. Proximal phalanx of digit V

16. Distal phalanx of digit V
17. Proximal sesamoid bones
18. Proximal phalanx of digit II
19. Middle phalanx of digit II
20. Distal phalanx of digit II
21. Greater trochanter of femur
22. Femur
23. Patella
24. Lateral fabella
25. Lateral femoral condyle
26. Fibula
27. Tarsal bones
28. Metatarsal bones
29. Phalanges

Figure 5-16, A
Type of animal: Chinchilla
Type of study: Stifle joint
Projection: Mediolateral
Weight of animal: 486 g
Gender: Male
Reproductive status: Intact
Age: Adult

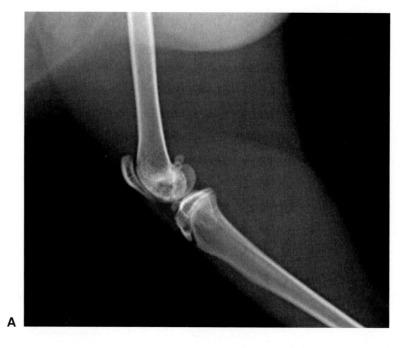

A

Figure 5-16, B
Type of animal: Chinchilla
Type of study: Stifle joint
Projection: Mediolateral
Weight of animal: 486 g
Gender: Male
Reproductive status: Intact
Age: Adult

1. Femur
2. Fabella
3. Fibula
4. Patella
5. Femoral condyles
6. Tibial tuberosity
7. Tibia

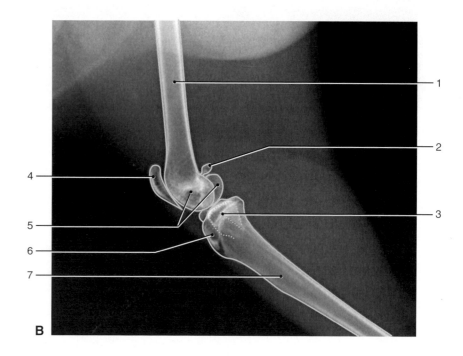

B

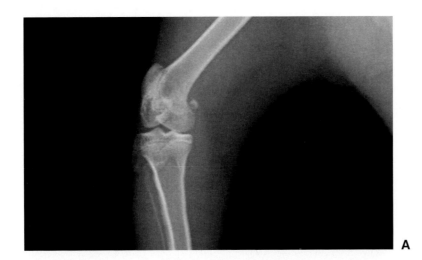

Figure 5-17, A
Type of animal: Chinchilla
Type of study: Stifle joint
Projection: Craniocaudal
Weight of animal: 486 g
Gender: Male
Reproductive status: Intact
Age: Adult

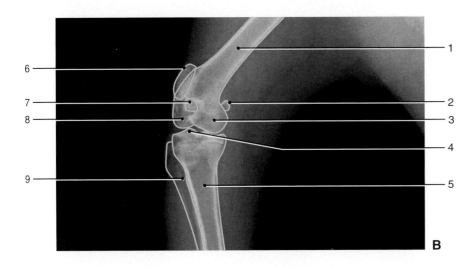

Figure 5-17, B
Type of animal: Chinchilla
Type of study: Stifle joint
Projection: Craniocaudal
Weight of animal: 486 g
Gender: Male
Reproductive status: Intact
Age: Adult

1. Femur
2. Medial fabella
3. Medial femoral condyle
4. Lateral tibial intercondylar tubercle
5. Tibia
6. Patella
7. Lateral fabella
8. Lateral femoral condyle
9. Fibula

Figure 5-18, A
Type of animal: Chinchilla
Type of study: Distal pelvic limb
Projection: Mediolateral
Weight of animal: 486 g
Gender: Male
Reproductive status: Intact
Age: Adult

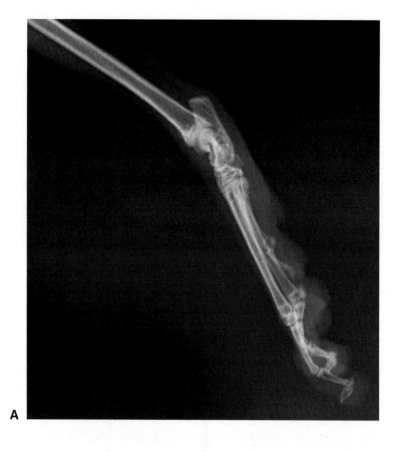

A

Figure 5-18, B
Type of animal: Chinchilla
Type of study: Distal pelvic limb
Projection: Mediolateral
Weight of animal: 486 g
Gender: Male
Reproductive status: Intact
Age: Adult

1. Tibia
2. Calcaneal tuber
3. Talus
4. Calcaneus
5. Medial tibial tarsal bone
6. Central tarsal bone
7. Tarsal bones I, II, III, and IV
8. Digit V
9. Proximal sesamoid bone
10. Metatarsal bone
11. Proximal phalanx
12. Middle phalanx
13. Distal phalanx
14. Trochlea of talus
15. Tarsal bones
16. Metatarsal bones
17. Phalanges

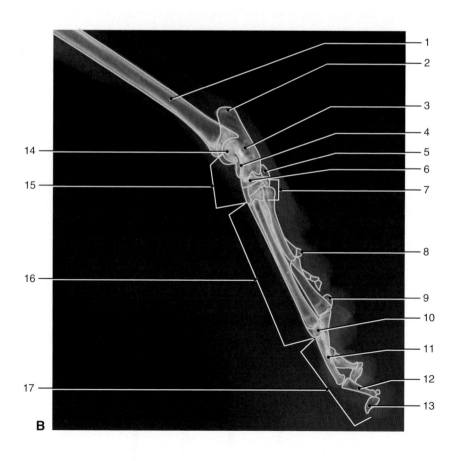

B

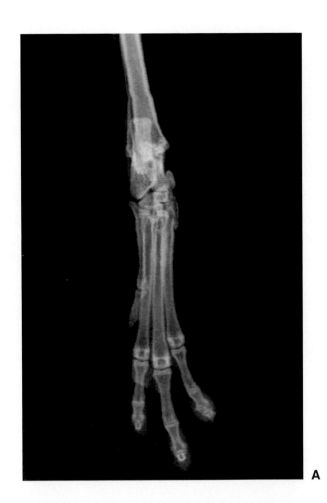

A

Figure 5-19, A
Type of animal: Chinchilla
Type of study: Distal pelvic limb
Projection: Dorsoplantar
Weight of animal: 486 g
Gender: Male
Reproductive status: Intact
Age: Adult

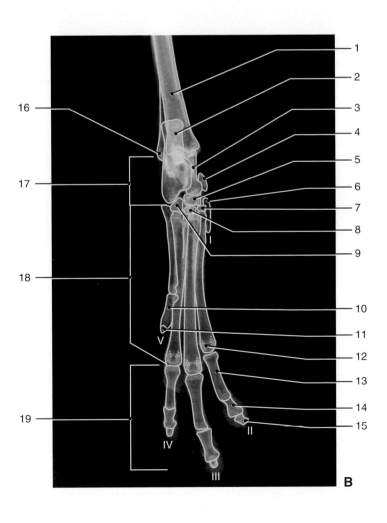

B

Figure 5-19, B
Type of animal: Chinchilla
Type of study: Distal pelvic limb
Projection: Dorsoplantar
Weight of animal: 486 g
Gender: Male
Reproductive status: Intact
Age: Adult

1. Tibia
2. Calcaneus
3. Talus
4. Medial tibial tarsal bone
5. Central tarsal bone
6. Tarsometatarsal bone I
7. Tarsal bone II
8. Tarsal bone III
9. Tarsal bone IV
10. Proximal phalanx of digit V
11. Distal phalanx of digit V
12. Proximal sesamoid bone
13. Proximal phalanx of digit II
14. Middle phalanx of digit II
15. Distal phalanx of digit II
16. Fibula
17. Tarsal bones
18. Metatarsal bones
19. Phalanges

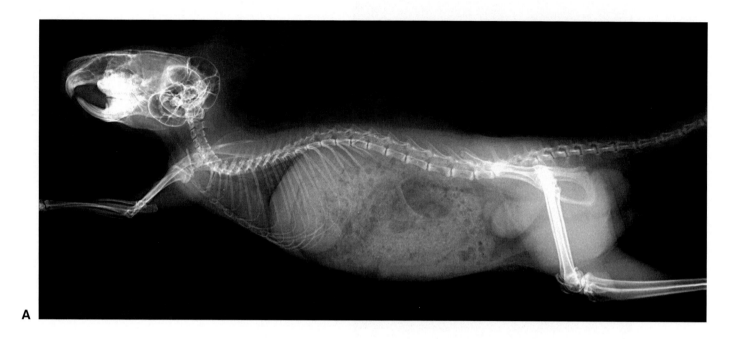

A

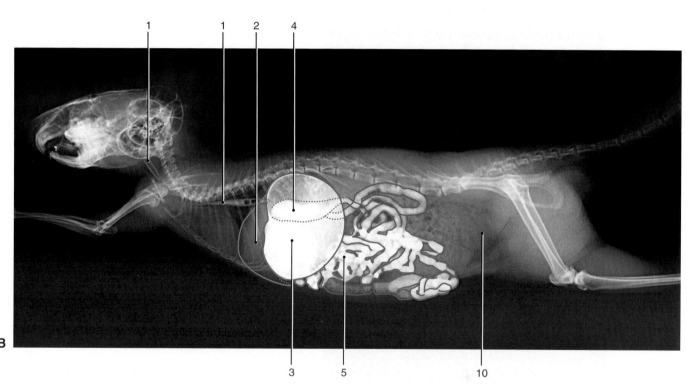

B

Figure 5-20, A-J
Type of animal: Chinchilla
Type of study: Gastrointestinal positive contrast study
Contrast medium: Barium sulfate suspension (Novopaque
   60% w/v; Lafayette Pharmaceutical, Inc., Lafayette, Ind.)
   12 ml administered per os
Projection: Laterolateral (right lateral recumbency)
Weight of animal: 480 g
Gender: Male
Reproductive status: Intact
Age: Adult

1. Esophagus
2. Liver
3. Stomach
4. Duodenum
5. Small intestine
6. Ileum
7. Cecum
8. Colon
9. Rectum
10. Urinary bladder

Image	Time (hr)
A	Survey
B	0.5

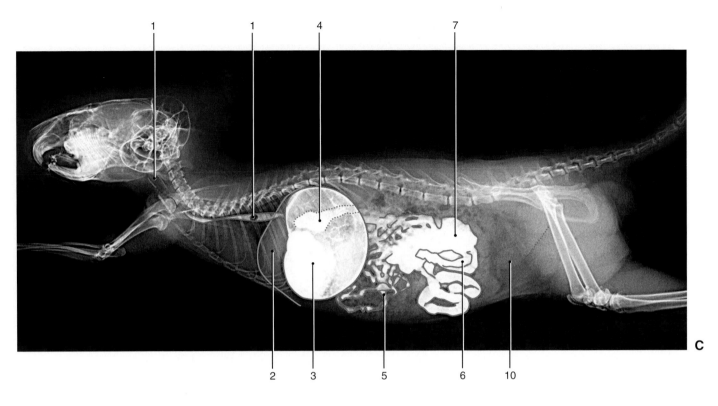

C

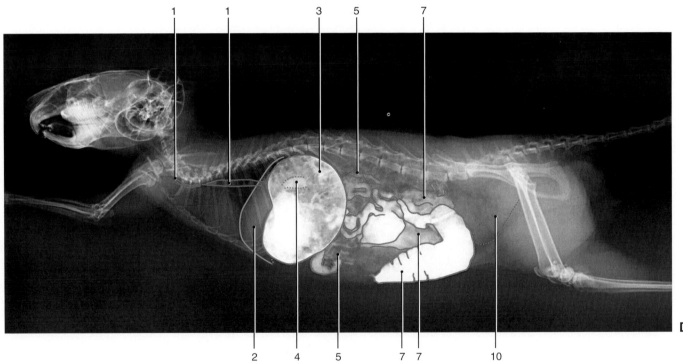

D

Figure 5-20, A-J—cont'd
Type of animal: Chinchilla
Type of study: Gastrointestinal positive contrast study
Contrast medium: Barium sulfate suspension (Novopaque
  60% w/v; Lafayette Pharmaceutical, Inc., Lafayette, Ind.)
  12 ml administered per os
Projection: Laterolateral (right lateral recumbency)
Weight of animal: 480 g
Gender: Male
Reproductive status: Intact
Age: Adult

1. Esophagus
2. Liver
3. Stomach
4. Duodenum
5. Small intestine
6. Ileum
7. Cecum
8. Colon
9. Rectum
10. Urinary bladder

Image	Time (hr)
C	1.0
D	2.0

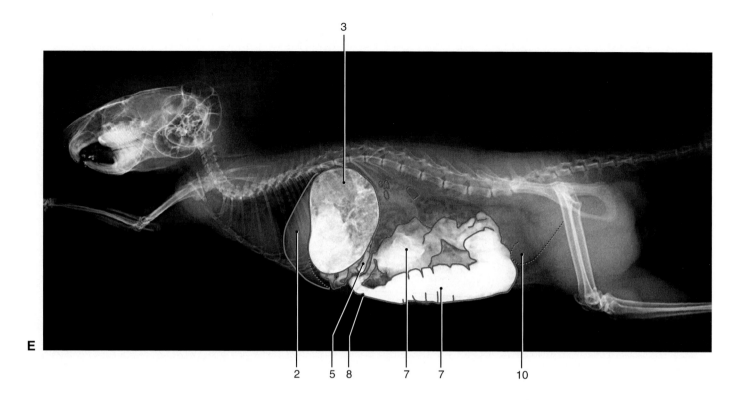

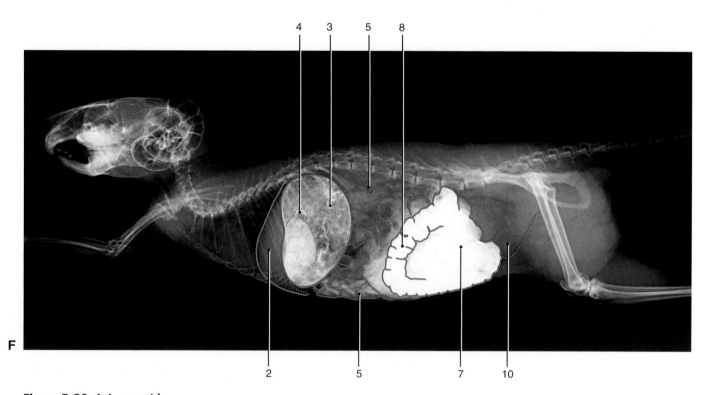

Figure 5-20, A-J—cont'd

Type of animal: Chinchilla
Type of study: Gastrointestinal positive contrast study
Contrast medium: Barium sulfate suspension (Novopaque
    60% w/v; Lafayette Pharmaceutical, Inc., Lafayette, Ind.)
    12 ml administered per os
Projection: Laterolateral (right lateral recumbency)
Weight of animal: 480 g
Gender: Male
Reproductive status: Intact
Age: Adult

1. Esophagus
2. Liver
3. Stomach
4. Duodenum
5. Small intestine
6. Ileum
7. Cecum
8. Colon
9. Rectum
10. Urinary bladder

Image	Time (hr)
E	3.5
F	5.5

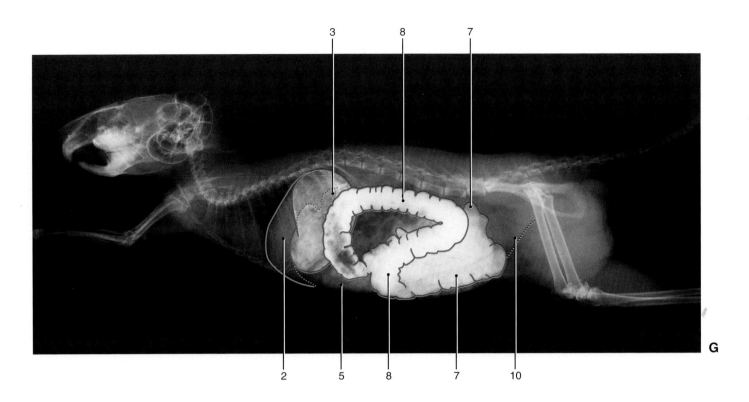

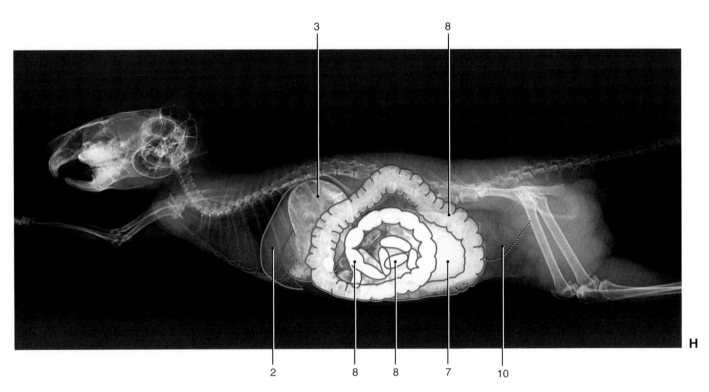

Figure 5-20, A-J—cont'd
Type of animal: Chinchilla
Type of study: Gastrointestinal positive contrast study
Contrast medium: Barium sulfate suspension (Novopaque
   60% w/v; Lafayette Pharmaceutical, Inc., Lafayette, Ind.)
   12 ml administered per os
Projection: Laterolateral (right lateral recumbency)
Weight of animal: 480 g
Gender: Male
Reproductive status: Intact
Age: Adult

1. Esophagus
2. Liver
3. Stomach
4. Duodenum
5. Small intestine
6. Ileum
7. Cecum
8. Colon
9. Rectum
10. Urinary bladder

Image	Time (hr)
G	7.5
H	9.5

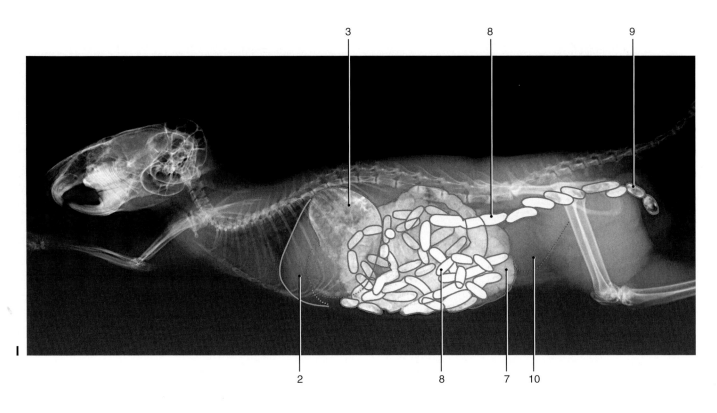

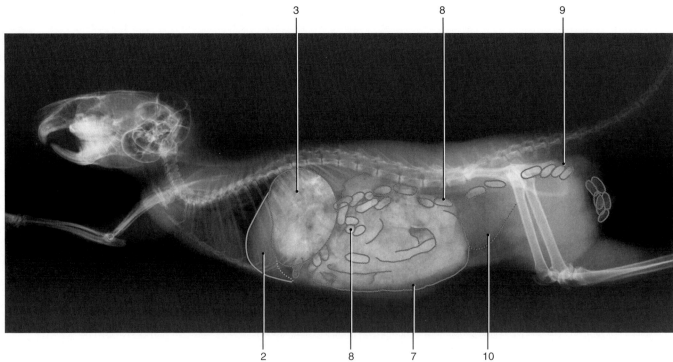

Figure 5-20, A-J—cont'd

Type of animal: Chinchilla
Type of study: Gastrointestinal positive contrast study
Contrast medium: Barium sulfate suspension (Novopaque
   60% w/v; Lafayette Pharmaceutical, Inc., Lafayette, Ind.)
   12 ml administered per os
Projection: Laterolateral (right lateral recumbency)
Weight of animal: 480 g
Gender: Male
Reproductive status: Intact
Age: Adult

1. Esophagus
2. Liver
3. Stomach
4. Duodenum
5. Small intestine
6. Ileum
7. Cecum
8. Colon
9. Rectum
10. Urinary bladder

Image	Time (hr)
I	14.5
J	24.0

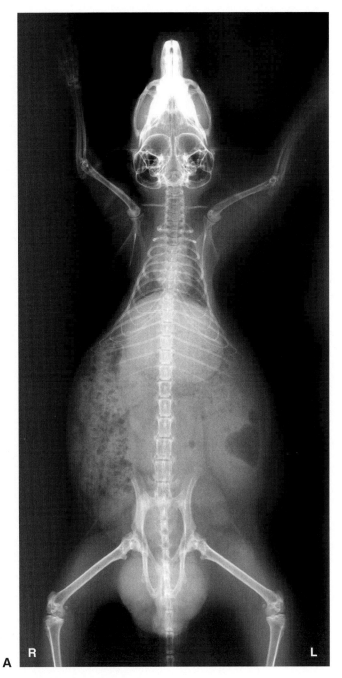

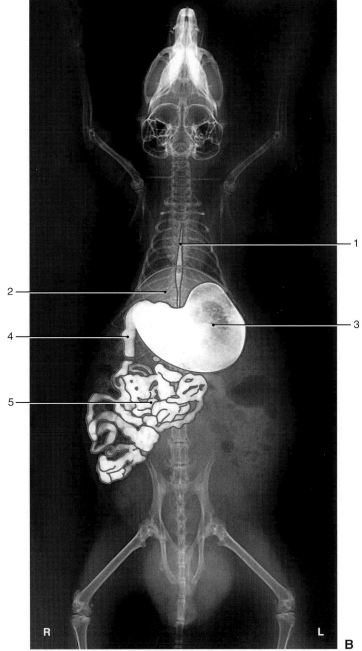

Figure 5-21, A-J
Type of animal: Chinchilla
Type of study: Gastrointestinal positive contrast study
Contrast medium: Barium sulfate suspension (Novopaque
 60% w/v; Lafayette Pharmaceutical, Inc., Lafayette, Ind.)
 12 ml administered per os
Projection: Ventrodorsal
Weight of animal: 480 g
Gender: Male
Reproductive status: Intact
Age: Adult

1. Esophagus
2. Liver
3. Stomach
4. Duodenum
5. Small intestine
6. Ileum
7. Cecum
8. Colon
9. Rectum
10. Urinary bladder

Image	Time (hr)
A	Survey
B	0.5

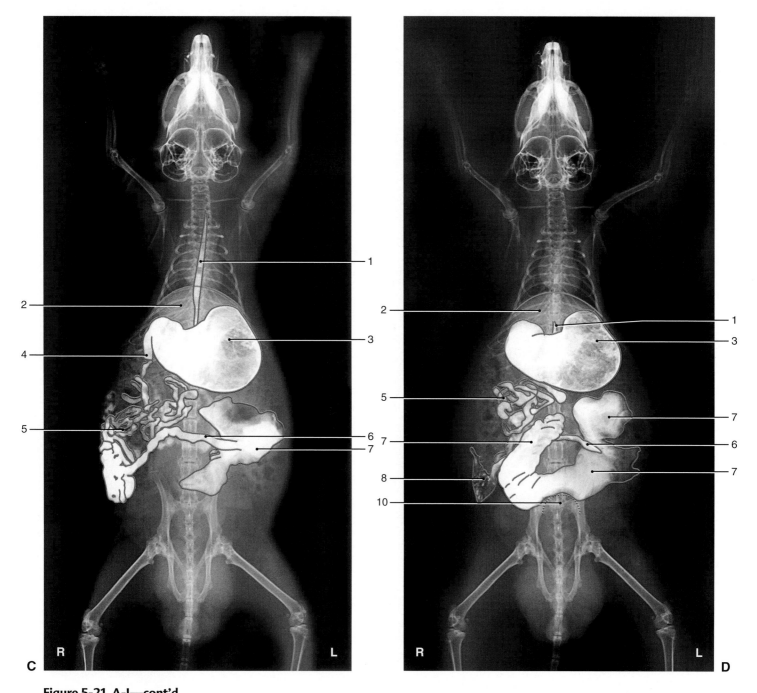

Figure 5-21, A-J—cont'd
Type of animal: Chinchilla
Type of study: Gastrointestinal positive contrast study
Contrast medium: Barium sulfate suspension (Novopaque
  60% w/v; Lafayette Pharmaceutical, Inc., Lafayette, Ind.)
  12 ml administered per os
Projection: Ventrodorsal
Weight of animal: 480 g
Gender: Male
Reproductive status: Intact
Age: Adult

1. Esophagus
2. Liver
3. Stomach
4. Duodenum
5. Small intestine
6. Ileum
7. Cecum
8. Colon
9. Rectum
10. Urinary bladder

Image	Time (hr)
C	1.0
D	2.0

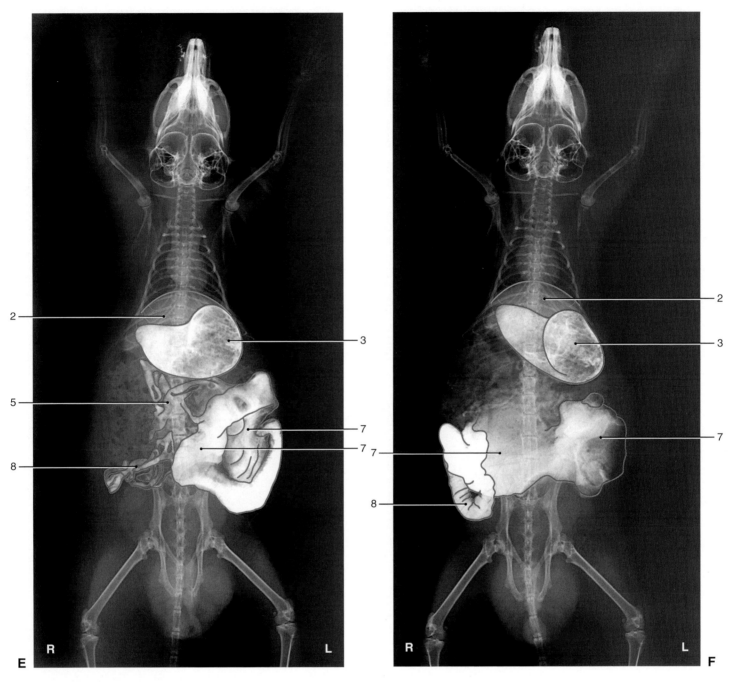

Figure 5-21, A-J—cont'd
Type of animal: Chinchilla
Type of study: Gastrointestinal positive contrast study
Contrast medium: Barium sulfate suspension (Novopaque
    60% w/v; Lafayette Pharmaceutical, Inc., Lafayette, Ind.)
    12 ml administered per os
Projection: Ventrodorsal
Weight of animal: 480 g
Gender: Male
Reproductive status: Intact
Age: Adult

1. Esophagus
2. Liver
3. Stomach
4. Duodenum
5. Small intestine
6. Ileum
7. Cecum
8. Colon
9. Rectum
10. Urinary bladder

Image	Time (hr)
E	3.5
F	5.5

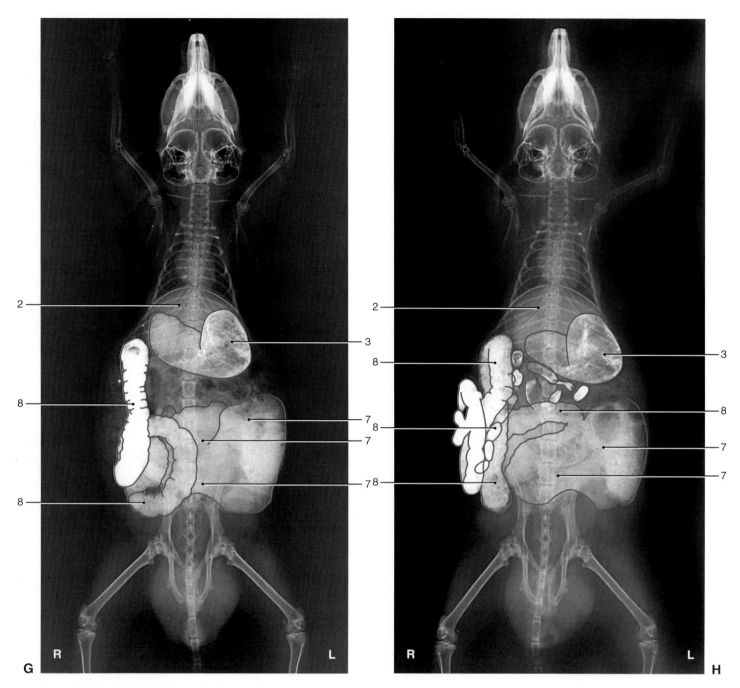

Figure 5-21—cont'd, A-J
Type of animal: Chinchilla
Type of study: Gastrointestinal positive contrast study
Contrast medium: Barium sulfate suspension (Novopaque 60% w/v; Lafayette Pharmaceutical, Inc., Lafayette, Ind.) 12 ml administered per os
Projection: Ventrodorsal
Weight of animal: 480 g
Gender: Male
Reproductive status: Intact
Age: Adult

1. Esophagus
2. Liver
3. Stomach
4. Duodenum
5. Small intestine
6. Ileum
7. Cecum
8. Colon
9. Rectum
10. Urinary bladder

Image	Time (hr)
G	7.5
H	9.5

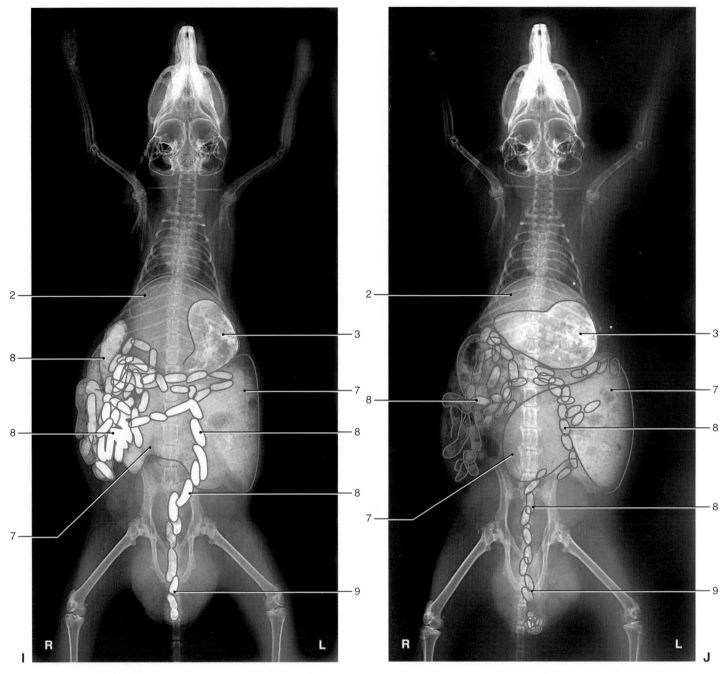

Figure 5-21—cont'd, A-J
Type of animal: Chinchilla
Type of study: Gastrointestinal positive contrast study
Contrast medium: Barium sulfate suspension (Novopaque
  60% w/v; Lafayette Pharmaceutical, Inc., Lafayette, Ind.)
  12 ml administered per os
Projection: Ventrodorsal
Weight of animal: 480 g
Gender: Male
Reproductive status: Intact
Age: Adult

1. Esophagus
2. Liver
3. Stomach
4. Duodenum
5. Small intestine
6. Ileum
7. Cecum
8. Colon
9. Rectum
10. Urinary bladder

Image	Time (hr)
I	14.5
J	24.0

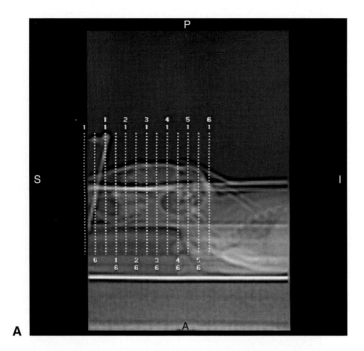

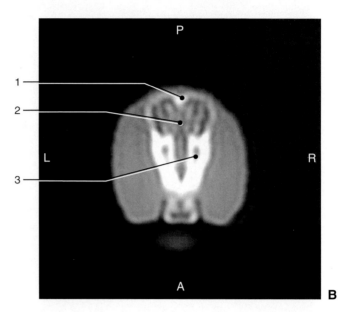

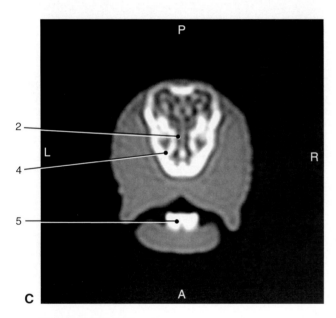

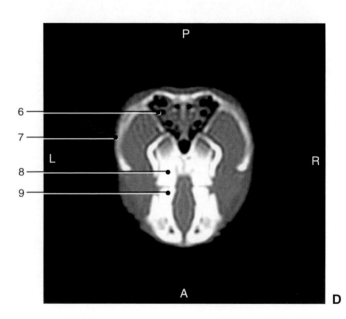

Figure 5-22, A-K
Type of animal: Chinchilla
Type of study: CT head
Imaging plane: Transverse
Weight of animal: 430 g
Gender: Male
Reproductive status: Intact
Age: Juvenile

1. Nasal bone
2. Nasal septum
3. Maxillary incisor tooth
4. Incisive bone
5. Mandibular incisor tooth
6. Nasoturbinates
7. Zygomatic bone
8. Maxillary molar tooth
9. Mandibular molar tooth
10. Frontal bone
11. Olfactory bulb

12. Frontal sinus
13. Maxilla
14. Nasal cavity
15. Mandible
16. Eyeball
17. Cerebrum
18. Nasopharynx
19. Parietal bone
20. Lens of eyeball
21. Mandibular ramus
22. Basisphenoidal bone

23. Temporomandibular joint
24. Condylar process of mandible
25. Tympanic cavity
26. Tympanic bulla
27. Hyoid bones
28. Larynx
29. Ear canal
30. Inner ear
31. Occipital bone
32. Cervical vertebra

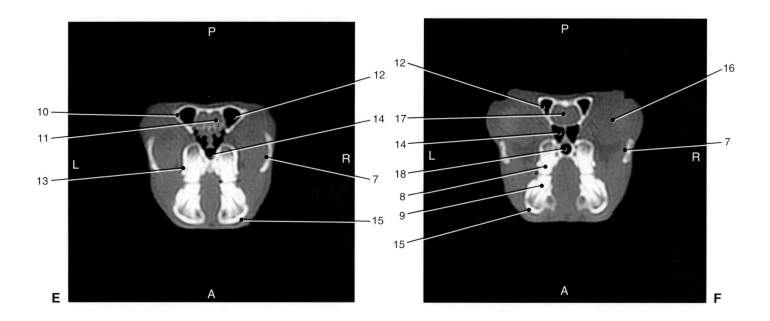

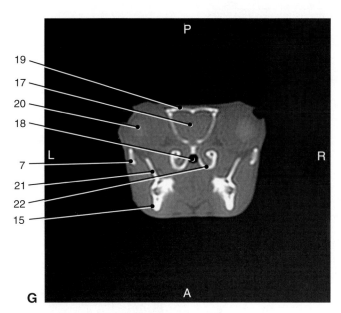

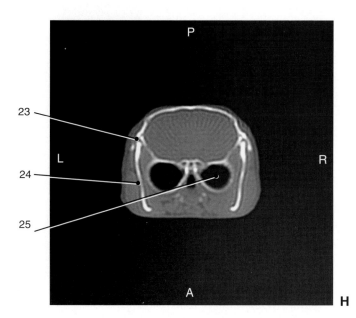

Figure 5-22—cont'd, A-K
Type of animal: Chinchilla
Type of study: CT head
Imaging plane: Transverse
Weight of animal: 430 g
Gender: Male
Reproductive status: Intact
Age: Juvenile

1. Nasal bone
2. Nasal septum
3. Maxillary incisor tooth
4. Incisive bone
5. Mandibular incisor tooth
6. Nasoturbinates
7. Zygomatic bone
8. Maxillary molar tooth
9. Mandibular molar tooth
10. Frontal bone
11. Olfactory bulb

12. Frontal sinus
13. Maxilla
14. Nasal cavity
15. Mandible
16. Eyeball
17. Cerebrum
18. Nasopharynx
19. Parietal bone
20. Lens of eyeball
21. Mandibular ramus
22. Basisphenoidal bone

23. Temporomandibular joint
24. Condylar process of mandible
25. Tympanic cavity
26. Tympanic bulla
27. Hyoid bones
28. Larynx
29. Ear canal
30. Inner ear
31. Occipital bone
32. Cervical vertebra

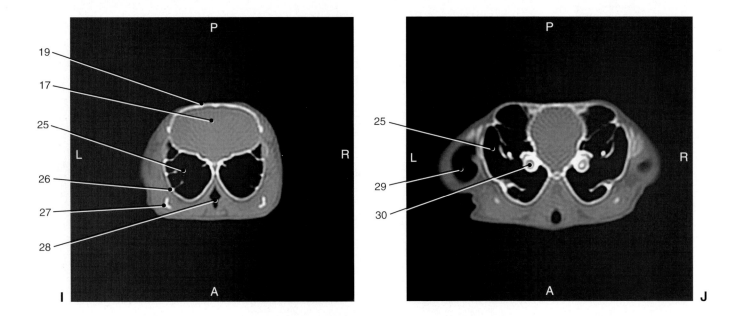

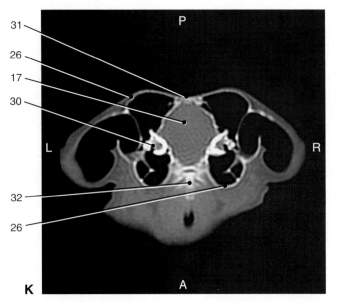

Figure 5-22—cont'd, A-K
Type of animal: Chinchilla
Type of study: CT head
Imaging plane: Transverse
Weight of animal: 430 g
Gender: Male
Reproductive status: Intact
Age: Juvenile

1. Nasal bone
2. Nasal septum
3. Maxillary incisor tooth
4. Incisive bone
5. Mandibular incisor tooth
6. Nasoturbinates
7. Zygomatic bone
8. Maxillary molar tooth
9. Mandibular molar tooth
10. Frontal bone
11. Olfactory bulb

12. Frontal sinus
13. Maxilla
14. Nasal cavity
15. Mandible
16. Eyeball
17. Cerebrum
18. Nasopharynx
19. Parietal bone
20. Lens of eyeball
21. Mandibular ramus
22. Basisphenoidal bone

23. Temporomandibular joint
24. Condylar process of mandible
25. Tympanic cavity
26. Tympanic bulla
27. Hyoid bones
28. Larynx
29. Ear canal
30. Inner ear
31. Occipital bone
32. Cervical vertebra

CHAPTER • 6

Domestic Guinea Pig (*Cavia porcellus*)

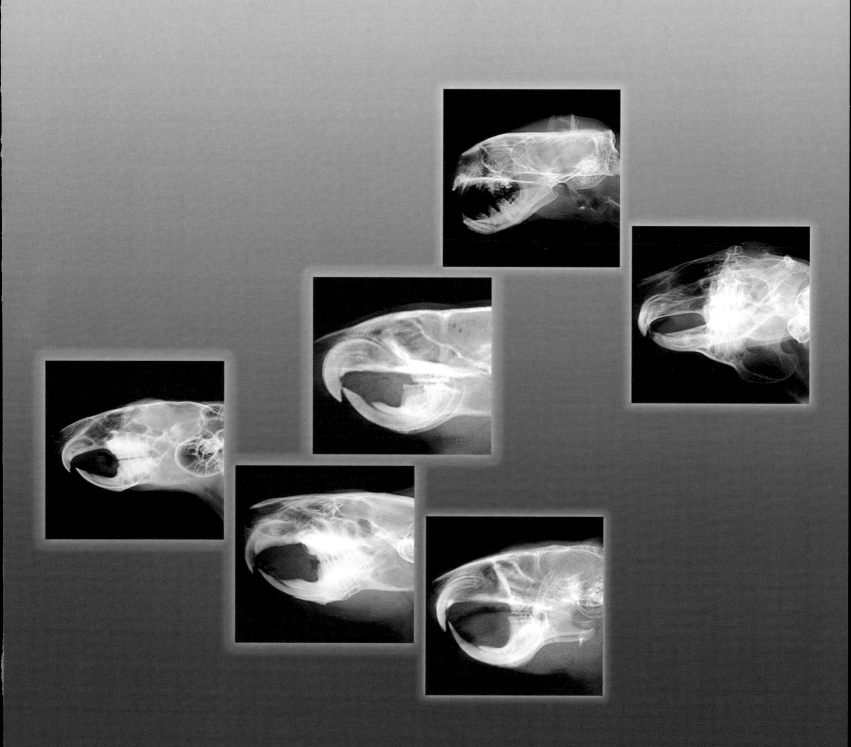

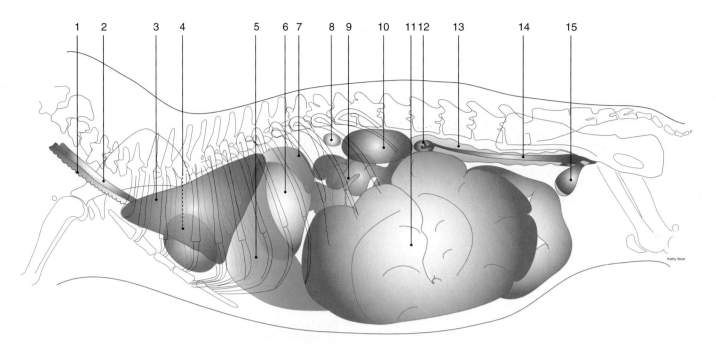

Figure 6-1, A Anatomic drawing (view of the left side) of viscera of the thorax and abdomen of an adult female guinea pig.

1. Trachea
2. Esophagus
3. Lung
4. Heart
5. Liver
6. Stomach
7. Spleen
8. Left adrenal gland
9. Small intestine
10. Left kidney
11. Cecum
12. Left ovary
13. Descending colon
14. Left horn of uterus
15. Urinary bladder

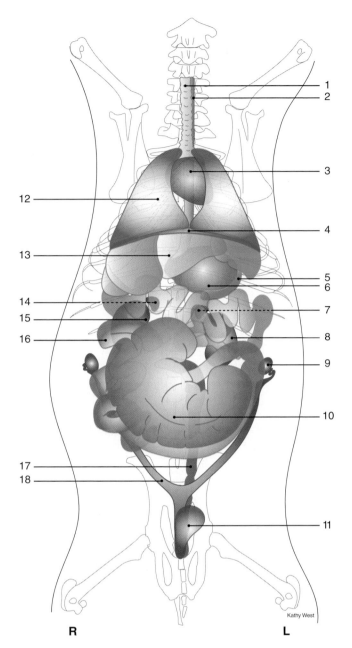

R   L

Kathy West

Figure 6-1, B Anatomic drawing (ventrodorsal view) of viscera of the thorax and abdomen of an adult female guinea pig.

1. Trachea
2. Esophagus
3. Heart
4. Diaphragm
5. Spleen
6. Stomach
7. Left adrenal gland
8. Left kidney
9. Left ovary
10. Cecum
11. Urinary bladder
12. Lung
13. Liver
14. Right adrenal gland
15. Right kidney
16. Small intestine
17. Descending colon
18. Right horn of uterus

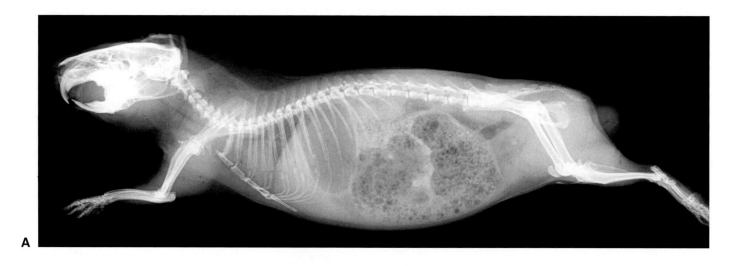

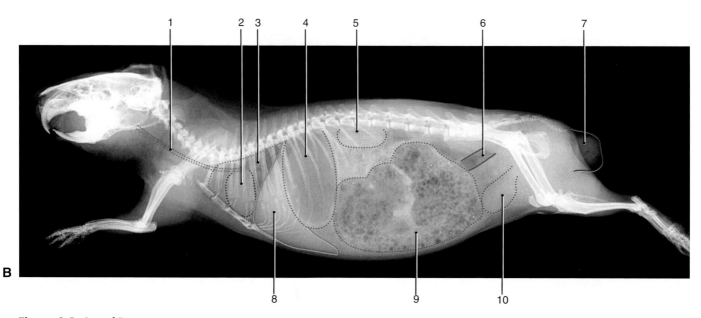

Figure 6-2, A and B
Type of animal: Guinea pig
Type of study: Viscera of thorax and abdomen
Projection: Laterolateral (right lateral recumbency)
Weight of animal: 1.2 kg
Gender: Male
Reproductive status: Intact
Age: 1.5 years

1. Trachea
2. Heart
3. Lung
4. Stomach
5. Kidney
6. Colon
7. Scrotum
8. Liver
9. Cecum
10. Urinary bladder

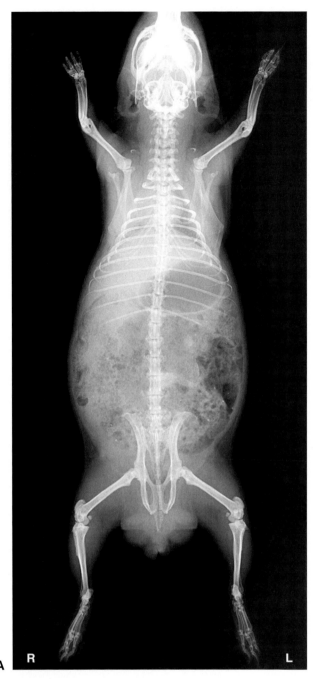

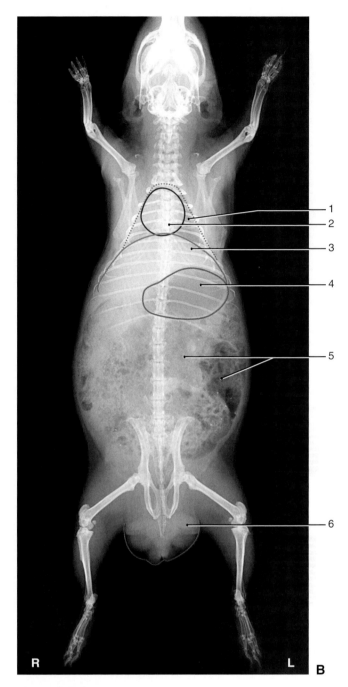

Figure 6-3, A
Type of animal: Guinea pig
Type of study: Viscera of thorax and abdomen
Projection: Ventrodorsal
Weight of animal: 1.2 kg
Gender: Male
Reproductive status: Intact
Age: 1.5 years

Figure 6-3, B
Type of animal: Guinea pig
Type of study: Viscera of thorax and abdomen
Projection: Ventrodorsal
Weight of animal: 1.2 kg
Gender: Male
Reproductive status: Intact
Age: 1.5 years

1. Lung
2. Heart
3. Liver
4. Stomach
5. Cecum
6. Scrotum

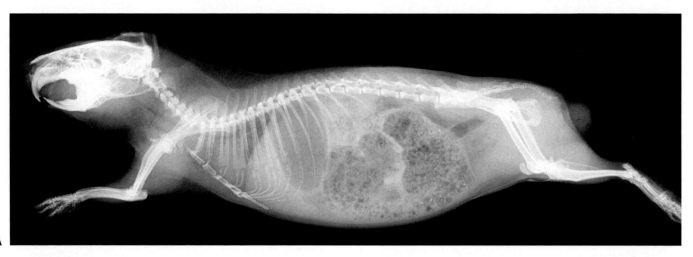

A

Figure 6-4, A
Type of animal: Guinea pig
Type of study: Whole body skeleton
Projection: Laterolateral (right lateral recumbency)
Weight of animal: 1.2 kg
Gender: Male
Reproductive status: Intact
Age: 1.5 years

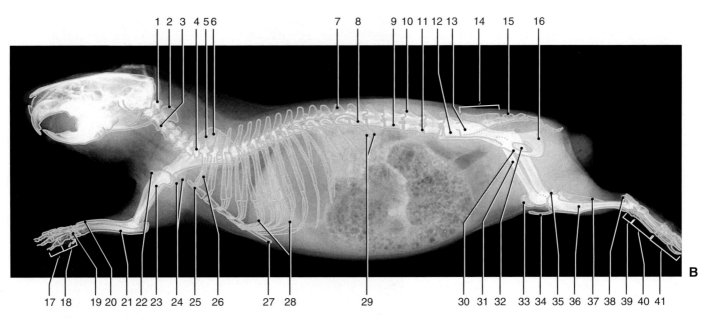

Figure 6-4, B
Type of animal: Guinea pig
Type of study: Whole body skeleton
Projection: Laterolateral (right lateral recumbency)
Weight of animal: 1.2 kg
Gender: Male
Reproductive status: Intact
Age: 1.5 years

1. Dorsal tubercle of atlas
2. Spinous process of axis
3. Cervical intervertebral space
4. 7th cervical vertebra
5. Spinous process of 1st thoracic vertebra
6. Scapula
7. Spinous process of 13th thoracic vertebra
8. 1st lumbar vertebra
9. Transverse process of lumbar vertebra
10. Spinous process of lumbar vertebra
11. Lumbar intervertebral space
12. 6th lumbar vertebra
13. Sacrum
14. Spinous processes of sacral vertebrae

15. Caudal vertebra
16. Ischium
17. Phalanges
18. Metacarpal bones
19. Carpal bone
20. Radius
21. Ulna
22. Clavicle
23. Humerus
24. Suprahamate processes
25. Manubrium of sternum
26. 1st rib
27. Xyphoid process
28. Costal cartilages
29. 13th ribs

30. Pubis
31. Femur
32. Obturator foramen
33. Patella
34. Os penis
35. Fabella
36. Tibia
37. Fibula
38. Calcaneus
39. Tarsal bones
40. Metatarsal bones
41. Phalanges

Figure 6-5, A
Type of animal: Guinea pig
Type of study: Whole body skeleton
Projection: Ventrodorsal
Weight of animal: 1.2 kg
Gender: Male
Reproductive status: Intact
Age: 1.5 years

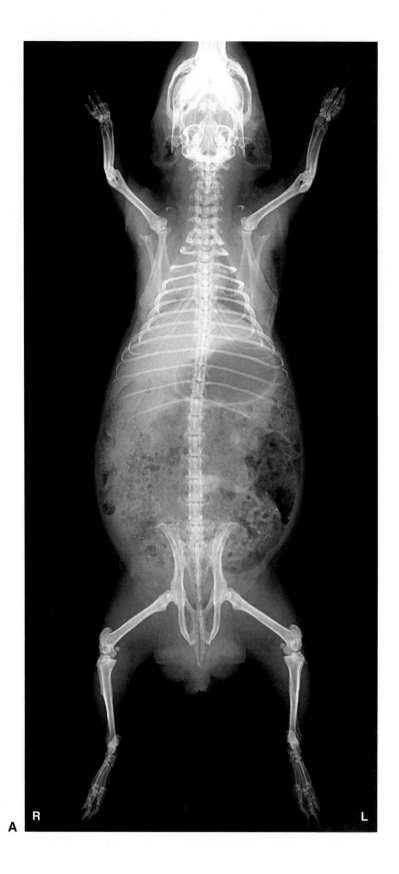

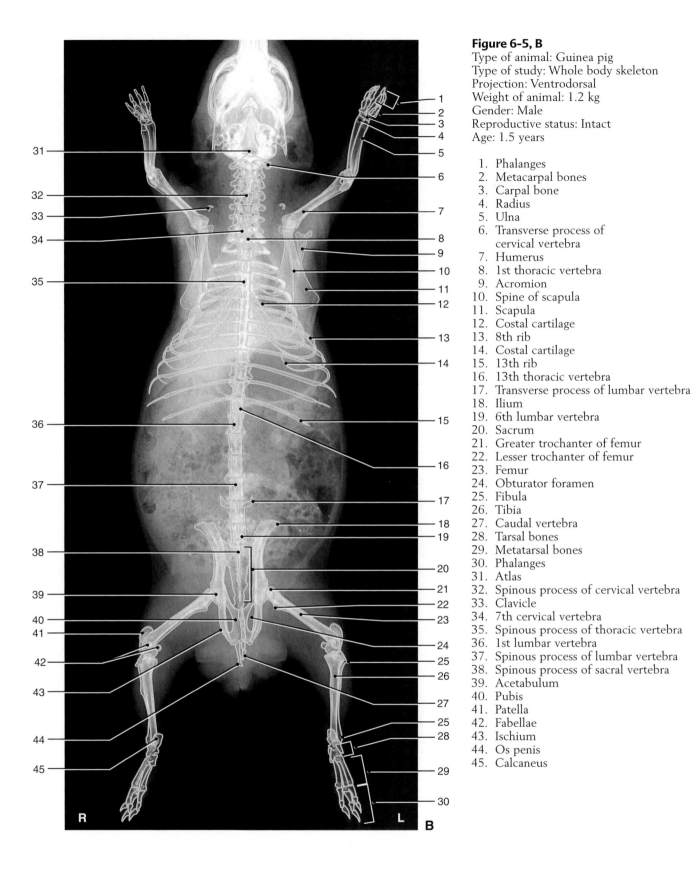

Figure 6-5, B
Type of animal: Guinea pig
Type of study: Whole body skeleton
Projection: Ventrodorsal
Weight of animal: 1.2 kg
Gender: Male
Reproductive status: Intact
Age: 1.5 years

1. Phalanges
2. Metacarpal bones
3. Carpal bone
4. Radius
5. Ulna
6. Transverse process of cervical vertebra
7. Humerus
8. 1st thoracic vertebra
9. Acromion
10. Spine of scapula
11. Scapula
12. Costal cartilage
13. 8th rib
14. Costal cartilage
15. 13th rib
16. 13th thoracic vertebra
17. Transverse process of lumbar vertebra
18. Ilium
19. 6th lumbar vertebra
20. Sacrum
21. Greater trochanter of femur
22. Lesser trochanter of femur
23. Femur
24. Obturator foramen
25. Fibula
26. Tibia
27. Caudal vertebra
28. Tarsal bones
29. Metatarsal bones
30. Phalanges
31. Atlas
32. Spinous process of cervical vertebra
33. Clavicle
34. 7th cervical vertebra
35. Spinous process of thoracic vertebra
36. 1st lumbar vertebra
37. Spinous process of lumbar vertebra
38. Spinous process of sacral vertebra
39. Acetabulum
40. Pubis
41. Patella
42. Fabellae
43. Ischium
44. Os penis
45. Calcaneus

Figure 6-6, A
Type of animal: Guinea pig
Type of study: Head
Projection: Laterolateral
    (right lateral recumbency)
Weight of animal: 1.2 kg
Gender: Male
Reproductive status: Intact
Age: Adult

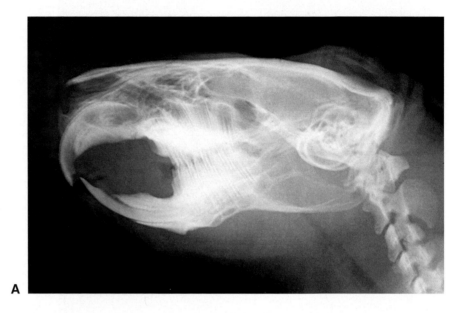

A

Figure 6-6, B
Type of animal: Guinea pig
Type of study: Head
Projection: Laterolateral
    (right lateral recumbency)
Weight of animal: 1.2 kg
Gender: Male
Reproductive status: Intact
Age: Adult

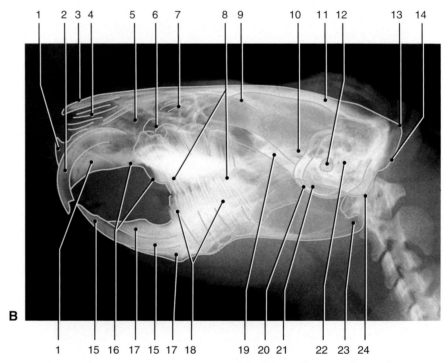

B

1. Incisive bone
2. Maxillary incisor tooth
3. Nasal bone
4. Nasoturbinates
5. Nasal cavity
6. Infraorbital hiatus
7. Ethmoturbinates
8. Maxillary premolar
    and molar teeth
9. Supraorbital margin
    of frontal bone
10. Temporal bone
11. Parietal bone
12. External acoustic meatus
13. External occipital protuberance
14. Occipital bone
15. Mandibular incisor tooth
16. Maxilla
17. Mandible
18. Mandibular premolar
    and molar teeth
19. Zygomatic bone
20. Tympanic bulla
21. Tympanic cavity
22. Petrous part of temporal bone
23. Angular process of mandible
24. Occipital condyle

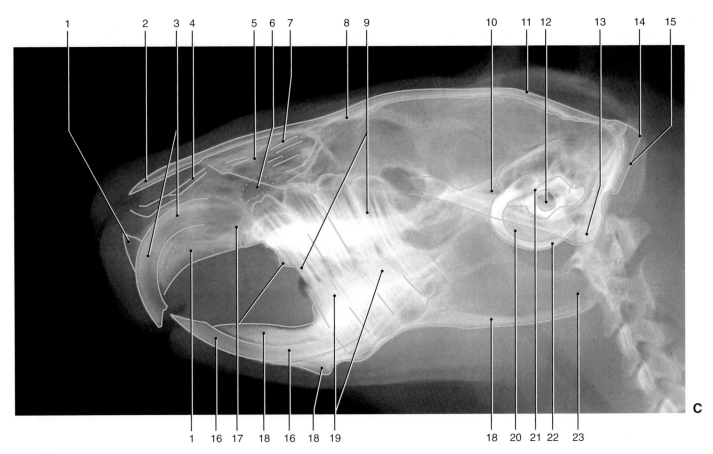

Figure 6-6, C
Type of animal: Guinea pig
Type of study: Magnification study of head
Projection: Laterolateral (right lateral recumbency)

1. Incisive bone
2. Nasal bone
3. Maxillary incisor tooth
4. Nasoturbinates
5. Nasal cavity
6. Infraorbital hiatus
7. Ethmoturbinates
8. Supraorbital margin of frontal bone
9. Maxillary premolar and molar teeth
10. Temporal bone
11. Parietal bone
12. External acoustic meatus
13. Occipital condyle
14. External occipital protuberance
15. Occipital bone
16. Mandibular incisor tooth
17. Maxilla
18. Mandible
19. Mandibular premolar and molar teeth
20. Tympanic cavity
21. Petrous part of temporal bone
22. Tympanic bulla
23. Angular process of mandible

Figure 6-7, A
Type of animal: Guinea pig
Type of study: Head
Projection: Oblique
 (30 degree) ventrodorsal
Weight of animal: 1.2 kg
Gender: Male
Reproductive status: Intact
Age: Adult

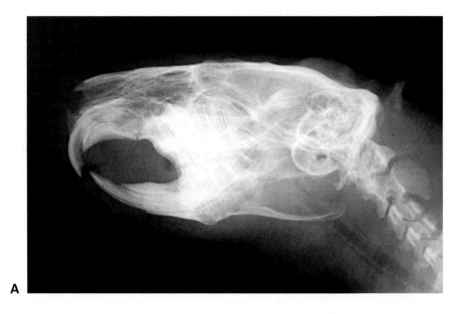

Figure 6-7, B
Type of animal: Guinea pig
Type of study: Head
Projection: Oblique
 (30 degree) ventrodorsal
Weight of animal: 1.2 kg
Gender: Male
Reproductive status: Intact
Age: Adult

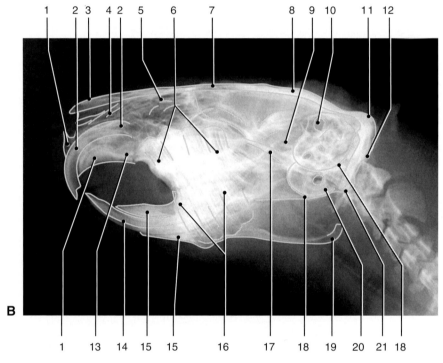

1. Incisive bone
2. Maxillary incisor tooth
3. Nasal bone
4. Nasoturbinates
5. Ethmoturbinates
6. Maxillary premolar
   and molar teeth
7. Frontal bone
8. Parietal bone
9. Temporal bone
10. External acoustic meatus
11. External occipital protuberance
12. Occipital bone
13. Maxilla
14. Mandibular incisor tooth
15. Mandible
16. Mandibular premolar
    and molar teeth
17. Zygomatic bone
18. Tympanic bulla
19. Angular process of mandible
20. Tympanic cavity
21. Occipital condyle

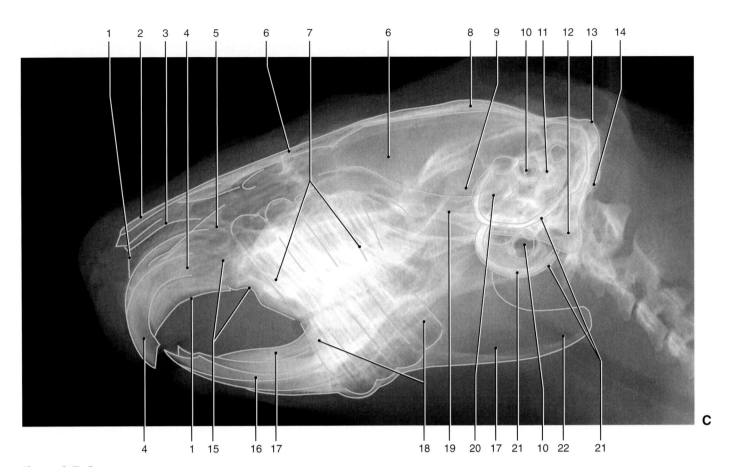

Figure 6-7, C
Type of animal: Guinea pig
Type of study: Magnification study of head
Projection: Oblique (30 degree) ventrodorsal

1. Incisive bone
2. Nasal bone
3. Nasoturbinates
4. Maxillary incisor tooth
5. Nasal cavity
6. Frontal bone
7. Maxillary premolar and molar teeth
8. Parietal bone
9. Temporal bone
10. External acoustic meatus
11. Petrous part of temporal bone
12. Occipital condyle
13. External occipital protuberance
14. Occipital bone
15. Maxilla
16. Mandibular incisor tooth
17. Mandible
18. Mandibular premolar and molar teeth
19. Zygomatic bone
20. Tympanic cavity
21. Tympanic bulla
22. Angular process of mandible

Figure 6-8, A
Type of animal: Guinea pig
Type of study: Head
Projection: Dorsoventral
Weight of animal: 1.2 kg
Gender: Male
Reproductive status: Intact
Age: Adult

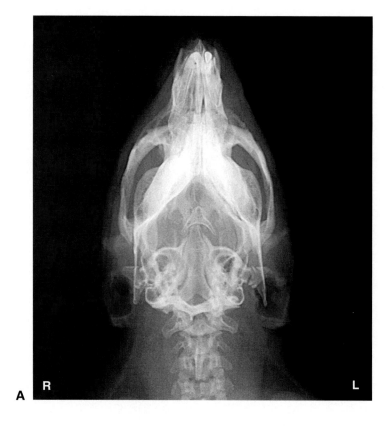

A   R   L

Figure 6-8, B
Type of animal: Guinea pig
Type of study: Head
Projection: Dorsoventral
Weight of Animal: 1.2 kg
Gender: Male
Reproductive status: Intact
Age: Adult

1. Incisive bone
2. Maxillary incisor tooth
3. Maxilla
4. Palatine bone
5. Mandible
6. Pterygoid bone
7. Tympanic cavity
8. Angular process of mandible
9. Paracondylar process of occipital bone
10. Foramen magnum
11. Nasal bone
12. Vomer
13. Infraorbital hiatus
14. Zygomatic process of maxilla
15. Zygomatic bone
16. Basisphenoidal bone
17. Rostral margin of pinna
18. Tympanic bulla
19. Ear canal
20. Occipital bone
21. Caudal margin of pinna
22. External occipital protuberance

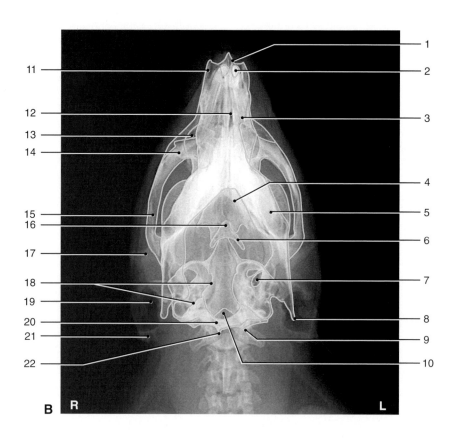

B   R   L

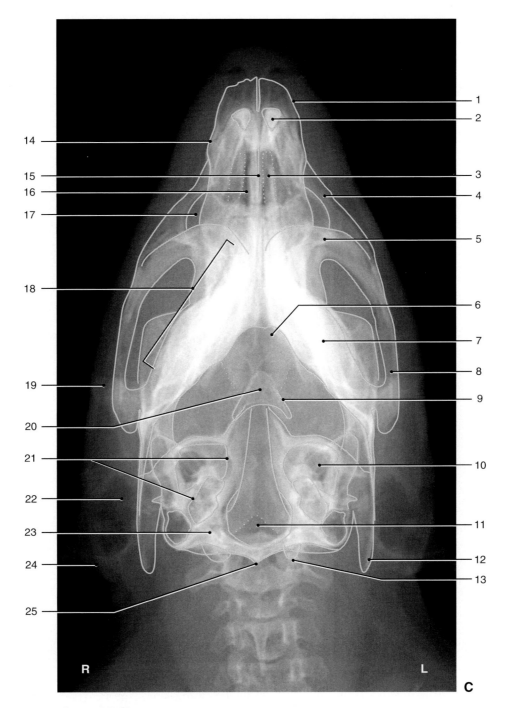

Figure 6-8, C
Type of animal: Guinea pig
Type of study: Magnification study of head
Projection: Dorsoventral

1. Nasal bone
2. Maxillary incisor tooth
3. Mandibular incisor tooth
4. Maxilla
5. Zygomatic process of maxilla
6. Palatine bone
7. Mandible
8. Zygomatic bone
9. Pterygoid bone
10. Tympanic cavity
11. Foramen magnum
12. Angular process of mandible
13. Paracondylar process of occipital bone
14. Incisive bone
15. Vomer
16. Nasal cavity
17. Infraorbital hiatus
18. Premolar and molar teeth
19. Rostral margin of pinna
20. Basisphenoidal bone
21. Tympanic bulla
22. Ear canal
23. Occipital bone
24. Caudal margin of pinna
25. External occipital protuberance

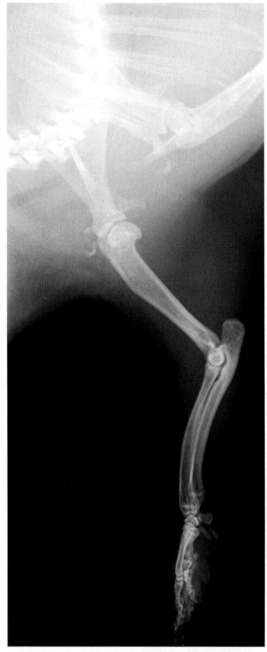

A

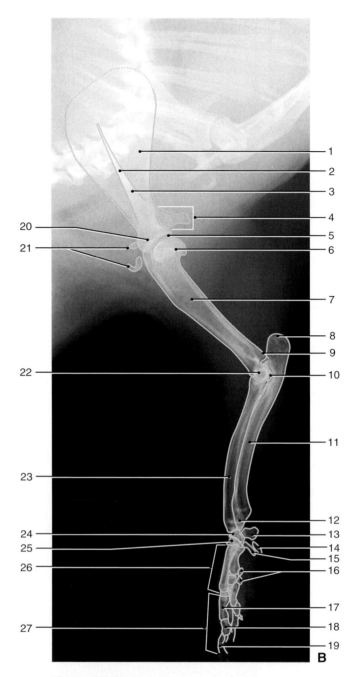

B

Figure 6-9, A
Type of animal: Guinea pig
Type of study: Thoracic limb
Projection: Mediolateral
Weight of animal: 1.2 kg
Gender: Male
Reproductive status: Intact
Age: 1.5 years

Figure 6-9, B
Type of animal: Guinea pig
Type of study: Thoracic limb
Projection: Mediolateral
Weight of animal: 1.2 kg
Gender: Male
Reproductive status: Intact
Age: 1.5 years

1. Scapula
2. Spine of scapula
3. Acromion
4. Hamate process
5. Scapulohumeral joint space
6. Humeral head
7. Humerus
8. Olecranon of ulna
9. Medial humeral epicondyle
10. Trochlear notch of ulna
11. Ulna
12. Styloid process of ulna
13. Accessory carpal bone
14. Falciform carpal bone
15. Metacarpal bone I
16. Proximal sesamoid bones
17. Proximal phalanx
18. Middle phalanx
19. Distal phalanx
20. Supraglenoid tubercle
21. Clavicle
22. Humeral condyle
23. Radius
24. Proximal row of carpal bones
25. Distal row of carpal bones
26. Metacarpal bones
27. Phalanges

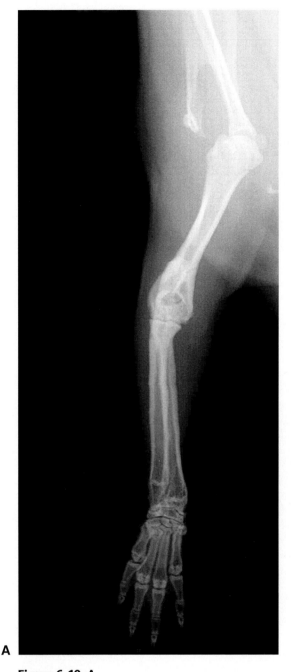

A

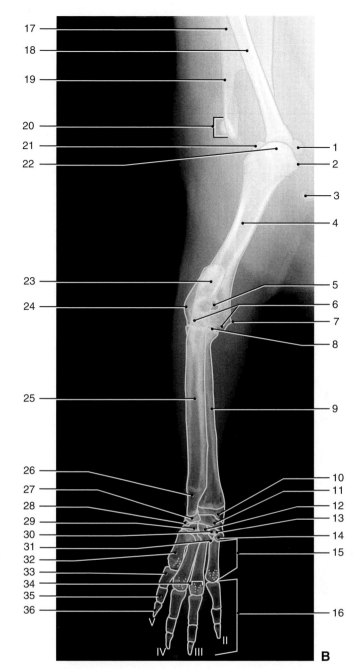

B

Figure 6-10, A
Type of animal: Guinea pig
Type of study: Thoracic limb
Projection: Ventrodorsal
Weight of animal: 1.2 kg
Gender: Male
Reproductive status: Intact
Age: 1.5 years

Figure 6-10, B
Type of animal: Guinea pig
Type of study: Thoracic limb
Projection: Ventrodorsal
Weight of animal: 1.2 kg
Gender: Male
Reproductive status: Intact
Age: 1.5 years

1. Coracoid process of scapula
2. Lesser tubercle of humerus
3. Clavicle
4. Humerus
5. Supratrochlear foramen of humerus
6. Humeral condyles
7. Medial humeral epicondyle
8. Humeroradial joint space
9. Radius
10. Distal radial epiphysis
11. Intermedioradial carpal bone
12. Carpal bone III

13. Carpal bone I
14. Metacarpal bone I
15. Metacarpal bones
16. Phalanges
17. Spine of scapula
18. Scapula
19. Acromion
20. Hamate and suprahamate processes
21. Greater tubercle of humerus
22. Humeral head
23. Olecranon of ulna
24. Lateral humeral epicondyle

25. Ulna
26. Styloid process of ulna
27. Ulnar carpal bone
28. Accessory carpal bone
29. Carpal bone IV
30. Carpal bone II
31. Falciform carpal bone
32. Metacarpal bone V
33. Proximal phalanx of digit V
34. Proximal sesamoid bones
35. Middle phalanx of digit V
36. Distal phalanx of digit V

Figure 6-11, A
Type of animal: Guinea pig
Type of study: Elbow joint
Projection: Mediolateral
Weight of animal: 1.2 kg
Gender: Male
Reproductive status: Intact
Age: 1.5 years

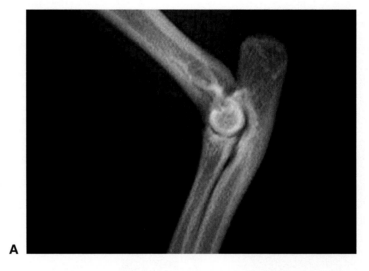

Figure 6-11, B
Type of animal: Guinea pig
Type of study: Elbow joint
Projection: Mediolateral
Weight of animal: 1.2 kg
Gender: Male
Reproductive status: Intact
Age: 1.5 years

1. Olecranon of ulna
2. Medial humeral epicondyle
3. Trochlear notch of ulna
4. Ulna
5. Humerus
6. Humeral condyle
7. Radius

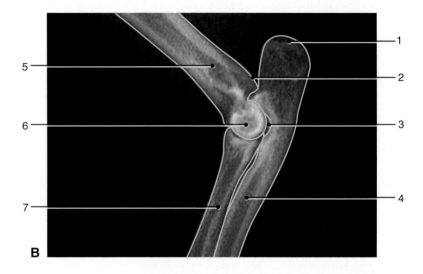

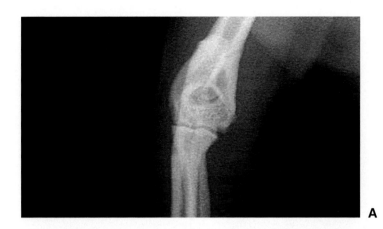

Figure 6-12, A
Type of animal: Guinea pig
Type of study: Elbow joint
Projection: Caudocranial
Weight of animal: 1.2 kg
Gender: Male
Reproductive status: Intact
Age: 1.5 years

A

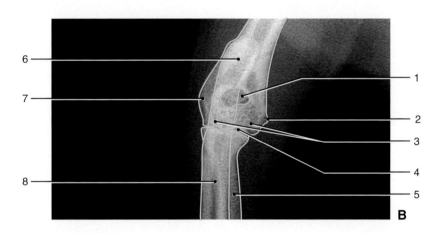

B

Figure 6-12, B
Type of animal: Guinea pig
Type of study: Elbow joint
Projection: Caudocranial
Weight of animal: 1.2 kg
Gender: Male
Reproductive status: Intact
Age: 1.5 years

1. Supratrochlear foramen of humerus
2. Medial humeral epicondyle
3. Humeral condyles
4. Humeroradial joint space
5. Radius
6. Olecranon of ulna
7. Lateral humeral epicondyle
8. Ulna

Figure 6-13, A
Type of animal: Guinea pig
Type of study: Distal thoracic limb
Projection: Mediolateral
Weight of animal: 1.2 kg
Gender: Male
Reproductive status: Intact
Age: 1.5 years

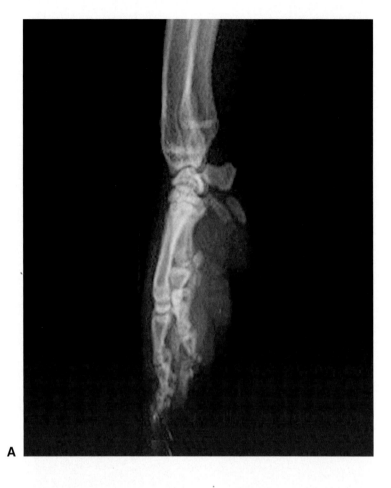

A

Figure 6-13, B
Type of animal: Guinea pig
Type of study: Distal thoracic limb
Projection: Mediolateral
Weight of animal: 1.2 kg
Gender: Male
Reproductive status: Intact
Age: 1.5 years

1. Ulna
2. Styloid process of ulna
3. Accessory carpal bone
4. Falciform carpal bone
5. Metacarpal bone I
6. Proximal sesamoid bones
7. Proximal phalanx
8. Middle phalanx
9. Distal phalanx
10. Radius
11. Proximal row of carpal bones
12. Distal row of carpal bones
13. Metacarpal bones
14. Phalanges

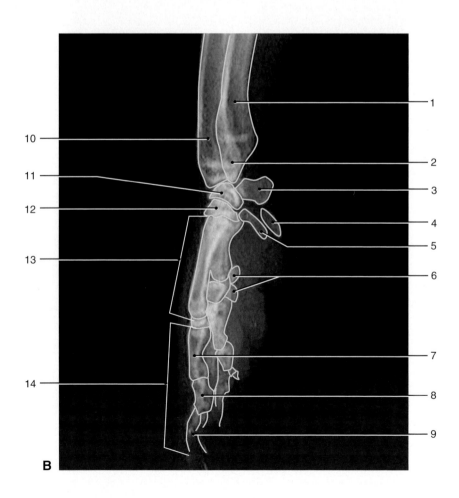

B

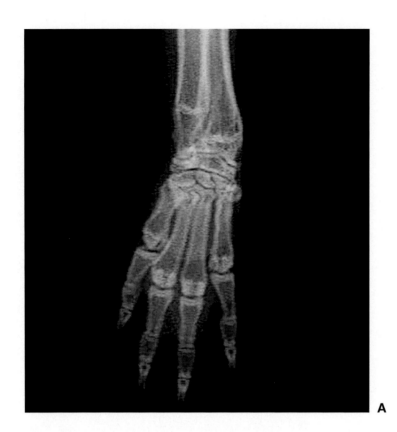

Figure 6-14, A
Type of Animal: Guinea pig
Type of Study: Distal thoracic limb
Projection: Dorsopalmar
Weight of animal: 1.2 kg
Gender: Male
Reproductive status: Intact
Age: 1.5 years

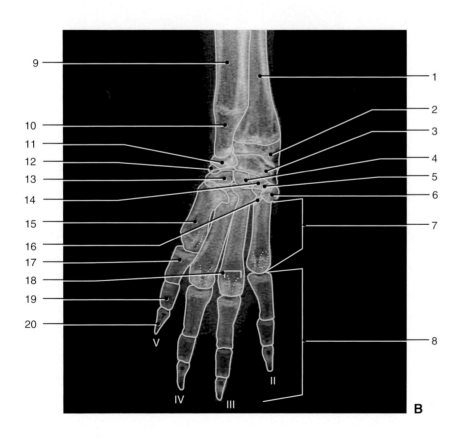

Figure 6-14, B
Type of animal: Guinea pig
Type of study: Distal thoracic limb
Projection: Dorsopalmar
Weight of animal: 1.2 kg
Gender: Male
Reproductive status: Intact
Age: 1.5 years

1. Radius
2. Distal radial epiphysis
3. Intermedioradial carpal bone
4. Carpal bone III
5. Carpal bone I
6. Metacarpal bone I
7. Metacarpal bones
8. Phalanges
9. Ulna
10. Styloid process of ulna
11. Ulnar carpal bone
12. Accessory carpal bone
13. Carpal bone IV
14. Carpal bone II
15. Metacarpal bone V
16. Falciform carpal bone
17. Proximal phalanx of digit V
18. Proximal sesamoid bones
19. Middle phalanx of digit V
20. Distal phalanx of digit V

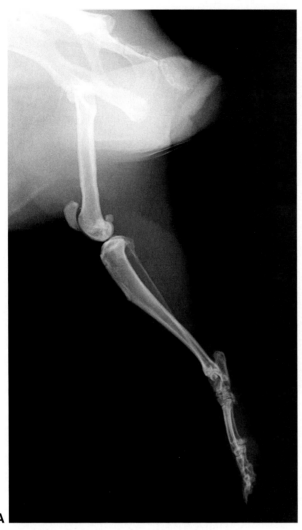

Figure 6-15, A
Type of animal: Guinea pig
Type of study: Pelvic limb
Projection: Mediolateral
Weight of animal: 1.2 kg
Gender: Male
Reproductive status: Intact
Age: 1.5 years

Figure 6-15, B
Type of animal: Guinea pig
Type of study: Pelvic limb
Projection: Mediolateral
Weight of animal: 1.2 kg
Gender: Male
Reproductive status: Intact
Age: 1.5 years

1. Greater trochanter of femur
2. Femur
3. Fabella
4. Fibula
5. Calcaneus
6. Talus
7. Middle row of tarsal bones
8. Distal row of tarsal bones
9. Tarsal bone II
10. Tarsometatarsal bone I
11. Metatarsal bone
12. Proximal sesamoid bones
13. Proximal phalanx
14. Middle phalanx
15. Distal phalanx
16. Femoral head
17. Patella
18. Femoral condyle
19. Tibia
20. Tarsal bones
21. Metatarsal bones
22. Phalanges

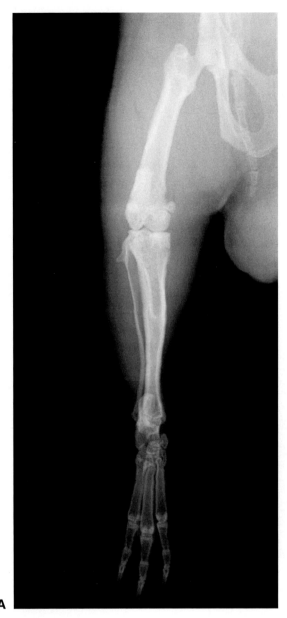

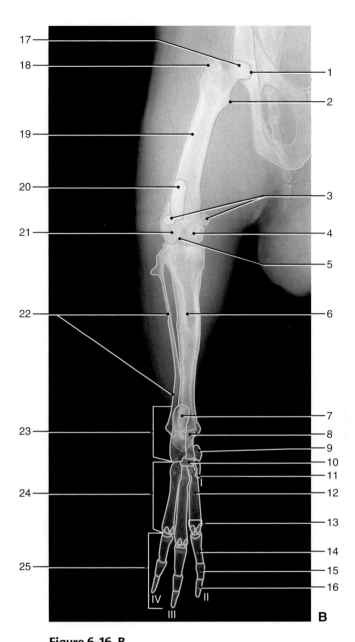

Figure 6-16, A
Type of animal: Guinea pig
Type of study: Pelvic limb
Projection: Ventrodorsal
Weight of animal: 1.2 kg
Gender: Male
Reproductive status: Intact
Age: 1.5 years

Figure 6-16, B
Type of animal: Guinea pig
Type of study: Pelvic limb
Projection: Ventrodorsal
Weight of animal: 1.2 kg
Gender: Male
Reproductive status: Intact
Age: 1.5 years

1. Acetabulum
2. Lesser trochanter of femur
3. Fabellae
4. Medial femoral condyle
5. Tibial intercondylar eminence
6. Tibia
7. Calcaneus
8. Talus
9. Medial tibial tarsal bone
10. Tarsal bone III
11. Tarsometatarsal bone I
12. Metatarsal bone II
13. Proximal sesamoid bones
14. Proximal phalanx of digit II
15. Middle phalanx of digit II
16. Distal phalanx of digit II
17. Femoral head
18. Greater trochanter of femur
19. Femur
20. Patella
21. Lateral femoral condyle
22. Fibula
23. Tarsal bones
24. Metatarsal bones
25. Phalanges

Figure 6-17, A
Type of animal: Guinea pig
Type of study: Stifle joint
Projection: Mediolateral
Weight of animal: 1.2 kg
Gender: Male
Reproductive status: Intact
Age: 1.5 years

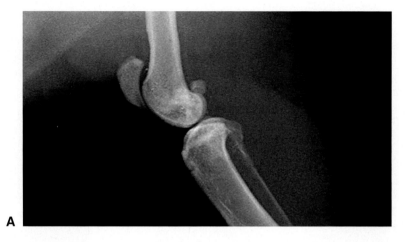

Figure 6-17, B
Type of animal: Guinea pig
Type of study: Stifle joint
Projection: Mediolateral
Weight of animal: 1.2 kg
Gender: Male
Reproductive status: Intact
Age: 1.5 years

1. Femur
2. Fabella
3. Fibula
4. Patella
5. Femoral condyle
6. Tibia

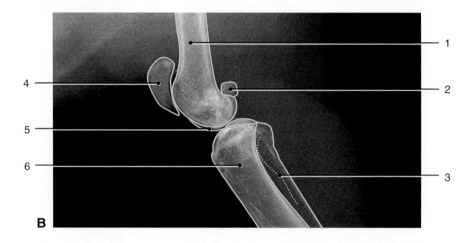

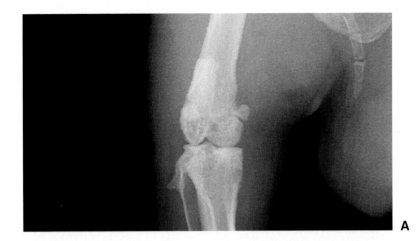

Figure 6-18, A
Type of animal: Guinea pig
Type of study: Stifle joint
Projection: Craniocaudal
Weight of animal: 1.2 kg
Gender: Male
Reproductive status: Intact
Age: 1.5 years

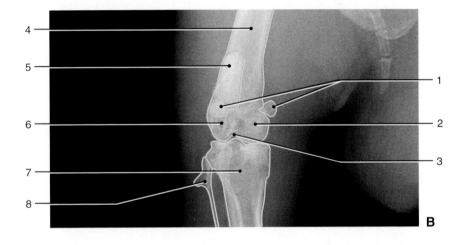

Figure 6-18, B
Type of animal: Guinea pig
Type of study: Stifle joint
Projection: Craniocaudal
Weight of animal: 1.2 kg
Gender: Male
Reproductive status: Intact
Age: 1.5 years

1. Fabellae
2. Medial femoral condyle
3. Tibial intercondylar eminence
4. Femur
5. Patella
6. Lateral femoral condyle
7. Tibia
8. Fibula

Figure 6-19, A
Type of animal: Guinea pig
Type of study: Distal pelvic limb
Projection: Mediolateral
Weight of animal: 1.2 kg
Gender: Male
Reproductive status: Intact
Age: 1.5 years

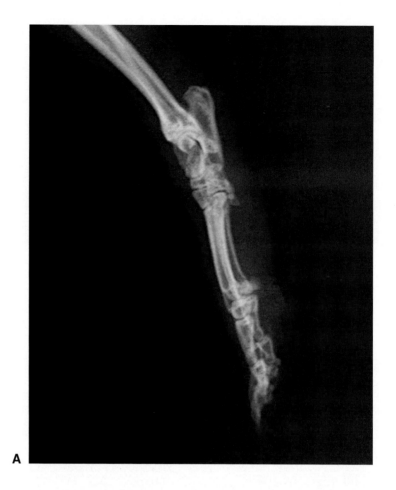

A

Figure 6-19, B
Type of animal: Guinea pig
Type of study: Distal pelvic limb
Projection: Mediolateral
Weight of animal: 1.2 kg
Gender: Male
Reproductive status: Intact
Age: 1.5 years

1. Calcaneus
2. Talus
3. Middle row of tarsal bones
4. Distal row of tarsal bones
5. Tarsal bone II
6. Tarsometatarsal bone I
7. Metatarsal bone
8. Proximal sesamoid bone
9. Proximal phalanx
10. Middle phalanx
11. Distal phalanx
12. Tibia
13. Tarsal bones
14. Metatarsal bones
15. Phalanges

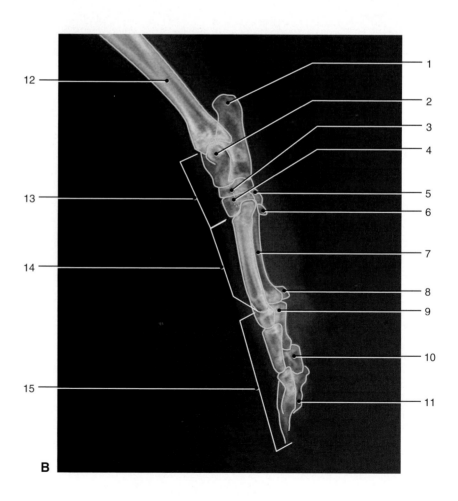

B

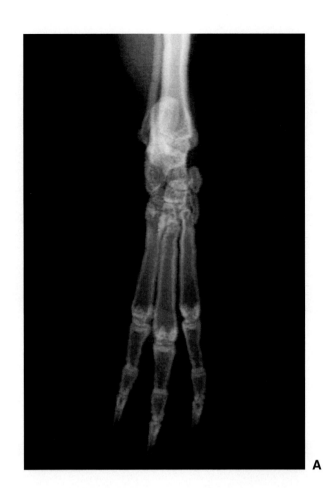

A

Figure 6-20, A
Type of animal: Guinea pig
Type of study: Distal pelvic limb
Projection: Dorsoplantar
Weight of animal: 1.2 kg
Gender: Male
Reproductive status: Intact
Age: 1.5 years

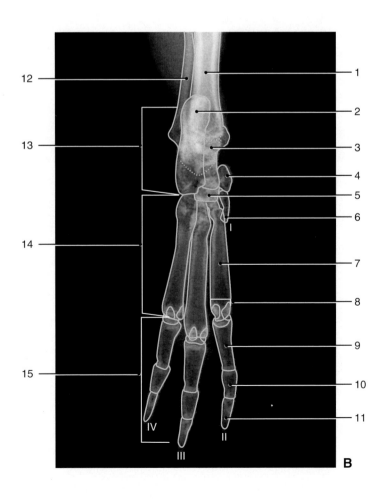

B

Figure 6-20, B
Type of animal: Guinea pig
Type of study: Distal pelvic limb
Projection: Dorsoplantar
Weight of animal: 1.2 kg
Gender: Male
Reproductive status: Intact
Age: 1.5 years

1. Tibia
2. Calcaneus
3. Talus
4. Medial tibial tarsal bone
5. Tarsal bone III
6. Tarsometatarsal bone I
7. Metatarsal bone II
8. Proximal sesamoid bones
9. Proximal phalanx of digit II
10. Middle phalanx of digit II
11. Distal phalanx of digit II
12. Fibula
13. Tarsal bones
14. Metatarsal bones
15. Phalanges

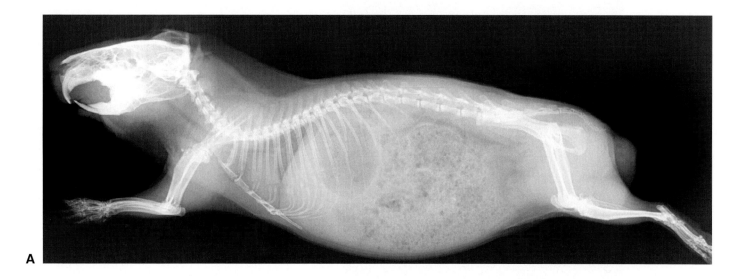

A

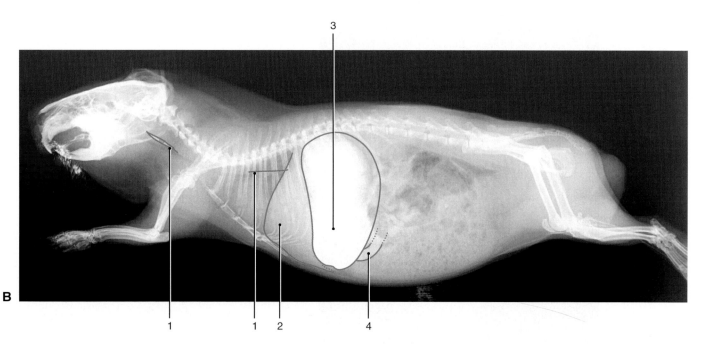

B

Figure 6-21, A-F

Type of animal: Guinea pig
Type of study: Gastrointestinal positive contrast study
Contrast medium: Barium sulfate suspension (Novopaque
    60% w/v; Lafayette Pharmaceutical, Inc., Lafayette, Ind.)
    30 ml administered per os
Projection: Laterolateral (right lateral recumbency)
Weight of animal: 1.2 kg
Gender: Male
Reproductive status: Intact
Age: Adult

1. Esophagus
2. Liver
3. Stomach
4. Duodenum
5. Small intestine
6. Cecum
7. Colon
8. Rectum
9. Urinary Bladder

Image	Time (hr)
A	Survey
B	0.25

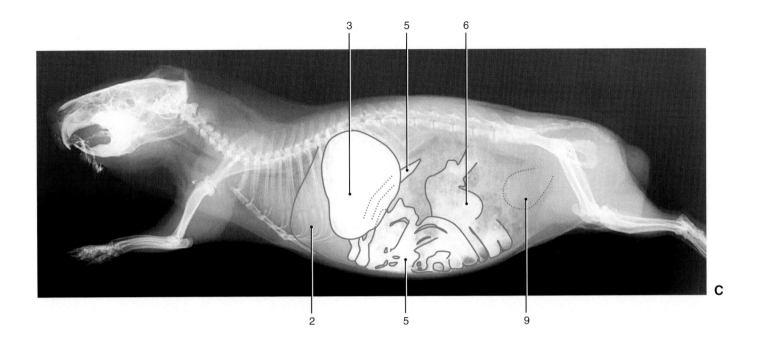

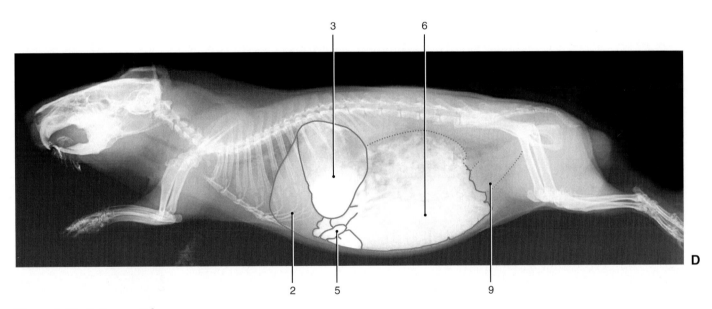

Figure 6-21, A-F—cont'd
Type of animal: Guinea pig
Type of study: Gastrointestinal positive contrast study
Contrast medium: Barium sulfate suspension (Novopaque
   60% w/v; Lafayette Pharmaceutical, Inc., Lafayette, Ind.)
   30 ml administered per os
Projection: Laterolateral (right lateral recumbency)
Weight of animal: 1.2 kg
Gender: Male
Reproductive status: Intact
Age: Adult

1. Esophagus
2. Liver
3. Stomach
4. Duodenum
5. Small intestine
6. Cecum
7. Colon
8. Rectum
9. Urinary Bladder

Image	Time (hr)
C	0.50
D	2.25

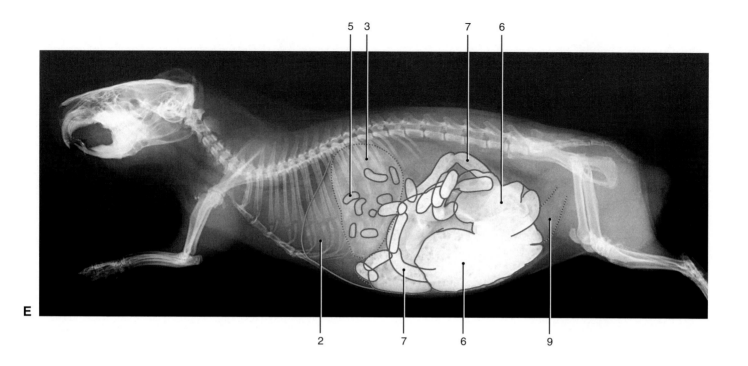

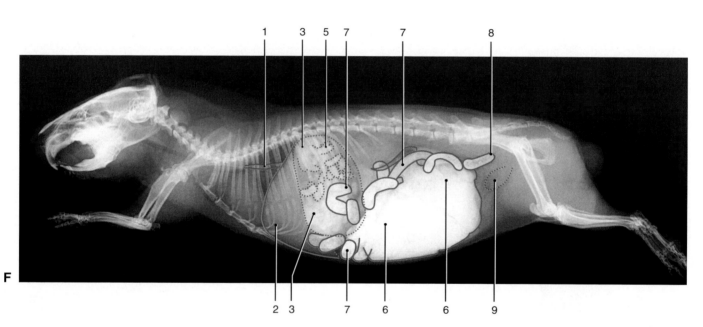

Figure 6-21, A-F—cont'd

Type of animal: Guinea pig
Type of study: Gastrointestinal positive contrast study
Contrast medium: Barium sulfate suspension (Novopaque
  60% w/v; Lafayette Pharmaceutical, Inc., Lafayette, Ind.)
  30 ml administered per os
Projection: Laterolateral (right lateral recumbency)
Weight of animal: 1.2 kg
Gender: Male
Reproductive status: Intact
Age: Adult

1. Esophagus
2. Liver
3. Stomach
4. Duodenum
5. Small intestine
6. Cecum
7. Colon
8. Rectum
9. Urinary Bladder

Image	Time (hr)
E	9.0
F	12.0

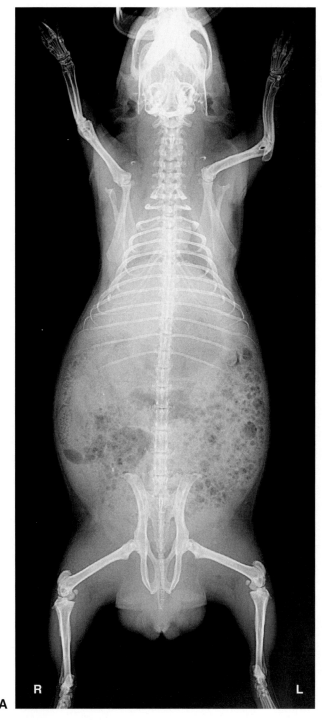

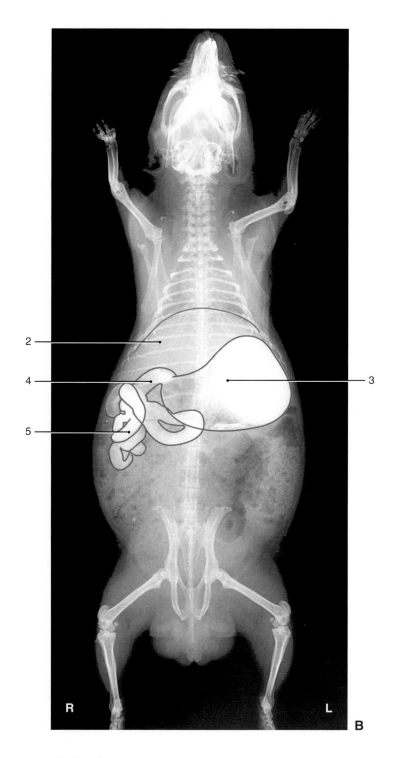

Figure 6-22, A-F
Type of animal: Guinea pig
Type of study: Gastrointestinal positive contrast study
Contrast medium: Barium sulfate suspension (Novopaque 60% w/v; Lafayette Pharmaceutical, Inc., Lafayette, Ind.) 30 ml administered per os
Projection: Ventrodorsal
Weight of animal: 1.2 kg
Gender: Male
Reproductive status: Intact
Age: Adult

1. Esophagus
2. Liver
3. Stomach
4. Duodenum
5. Small intestine
6. Cecum
7. Colon
8. Rectum
9. Urinary bladder

Image	Time (hr)
A	Survey
B	0.25

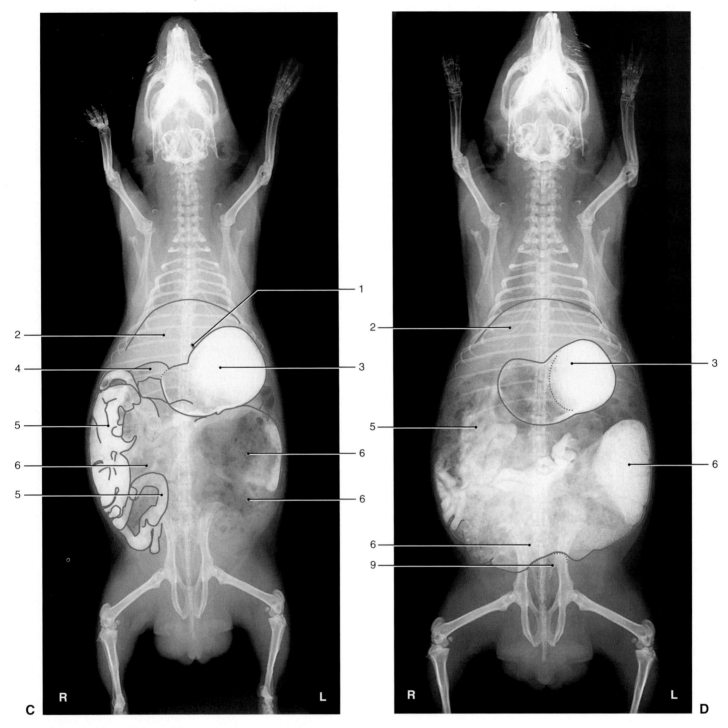

Figure 6-22, A-F—cont'd
Type of animal: Guinea pig
Type of study: Gastrointestinal positive contrast study
Contrast medium: Barium sulfate suspension (Novopaque
   60% w/v; Lafayette Pharmaceutical, Inc., Lafayette, Ind.)
   30 ml administered per os
Projection: Ventrodorsal
Weight of animal: 1.2 kg
Gender: Male
Reproductive status: Intact
Age: Adult

1. Esophagus
2. Liver
3. Stomach
4. Duodenum
5. Small intestine
6. Cecum
7. Colon
8. Rectum
9. Urinary bladder

Image	Time (hr)
C	0.50
D	2.25

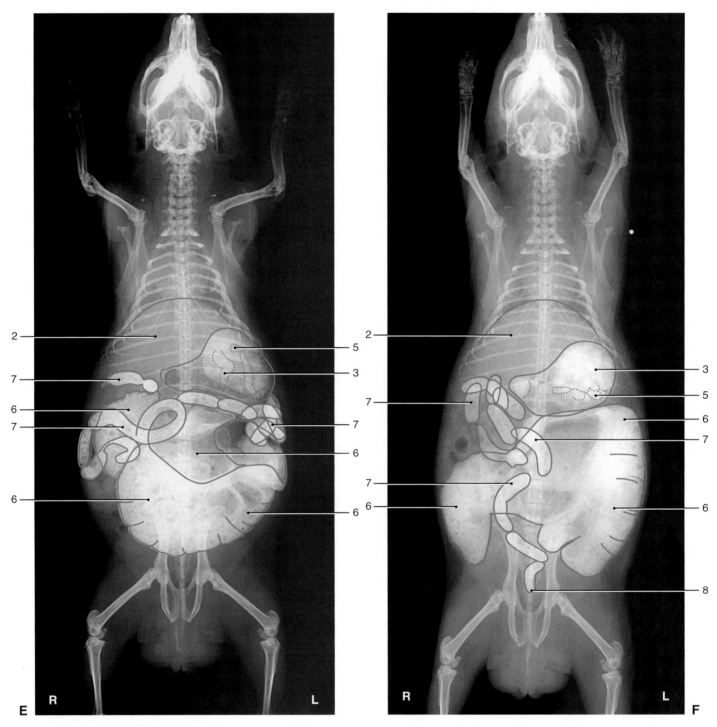

Figure 6-22, A-F—cont'd
Type of animal: Guinea pig
Type of study: Gastrointestinal positive contrast study
Contrast medium: Barium sulfate suspension (Novopaque 60% w/v; Lafayette Pharmaceutical, Inc., Lafayette, Ind.) 30 ml administered per os
Projection: Ventrodorsal
Weight of animal: 1.2 kg
Gender: Male
Reproductive status: Intact
Age: Adult

1. Esophagus
2. Liver
3. Stomach
4. Duodenum
5. Small intestine
6. Cecum
7. Colon
8. Rectum
9. Urinary bladder

Image	Time (hr)
E	9.00
F	12.00

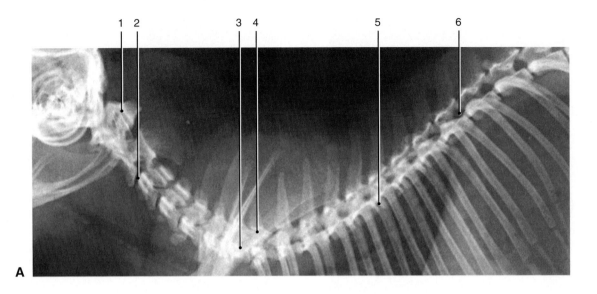

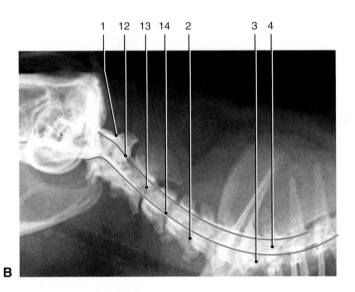

Figure 6-23, A-G

Type of animal: Guinea pig
Type of study: Myelogram
Contrast medium: Isovue 200 (iopamidol injection 41%, 20% bound iodine; Bracco Diagnostics, Inc., Princeton, NJ); injection site L6-S1
Projection: Laterolateral (right lateral recumbency)
Weight of animal: 1.2 kg
Gender: Male
Reproductive status: Intact
Age: Adult

Image	Projection
A	Cervico-thoracic vertebral column survey
B	Cervical vertebral column myelogram

1. Atlas
2. Cervical intervertebral space
3. 7th cervical vertebra
4. 1st thoracic vertebra
5. Thoracic intervertebral space
6. Thoracic intervertebral foramen
7. 13th thoracic vertebra
8. 1st lumbar vertebra
9. Lumbar intervertebral space
10. Lumbar intervertebral foramen
11. 6th lumbar vertebra
12. Dorsal aspect of subarachnoid space
13. Spinal cord
14. Ventral aspect of subarachnoid space
15. Spinal needle

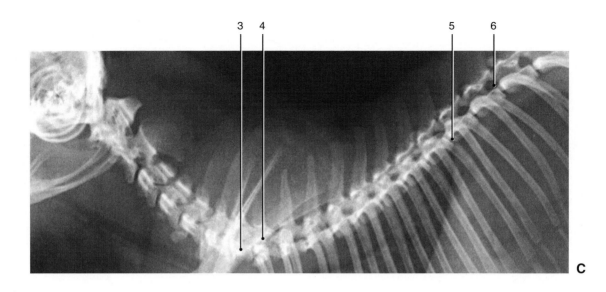

C

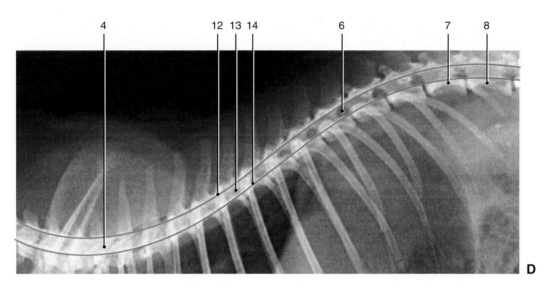

D

Figure 6-23, A-G—cont'd
Type of animal: Guinea pig
Type of study: Myelogram
Contrast medium: Isovue 200 (iopamidol injection 41%,
 20% bound iodine; Bracco Diagnostics, Inc., Princeton,
 NJ); injection site L6-S1
Projection: Laterolateral (right lateral recumbency)
Weight of animal: 1.2 kg
Gender: Male
Reproductive status: Intact
Age: Adult

Image	Projection
C	Cervico-thoracic column survey
D	Thoracic vertebral column myelogram

1. Atlas
2. Cervical intervertebral space
3. 7th cervical vertebra
4. 1st thoracic vertebra
5. Thoracic intervertebral space
6. Thoracic intervertebral foramen
7. 13th thoracic vertebra
8. 1st lumbar vertebra
9. Lumbar intervertebral space
10. Lumbar intervertebral foramen
11. 6th lumbar vertebra
12. Dorsal aspect of subarachnoid space
13. Spinal cord
14. Ventral aspect of subarachnoid space
15. Spinal needle

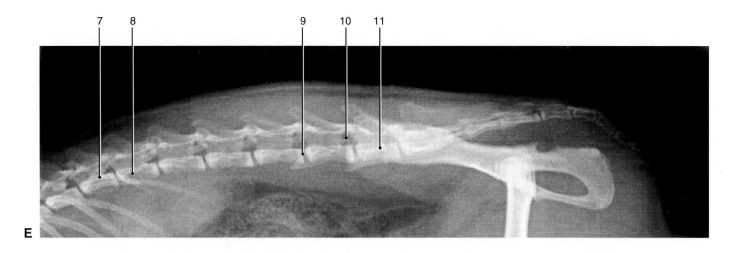

E

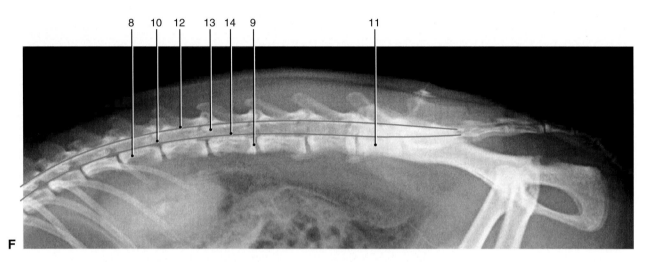

F

Figure 6-23, A-G—cont'd

Type of animal: Guinea pig
Type of study: Myelogram
Contrast medium: Isovue 200 (iopamidol injection 41%,
   20% bound iodine; Bracco Diagnostics, Inc., Princeton,
   NJ); injection site L6-S1
Projection: Laterolateral (right lateral recumbency)
Weight of animal: 1.2 kg
Gender: Male
Reproductive status: Intact
Age: Adult

1. Atlas
2. Cervical intervertebral space
3. 7th cervical vertebra
4. 1st thoracic vertebra
5. Thoracic intervertebral space
6. Thoracic intervertebral foramen
7. 13th thoracic vertebra
8. 1st lumbar vertebra
9. Lumbar intervertebral space
10. Lumbar intervertebral foramen
11. 6th lumbar vertebra
12. Dorsal aspect of subarachnoid space
13. Spinal cord
14. Ventral aspect of subarachnoid space
15. Spinal needle

Image	Projection
E	Lumbar vertebral column survey
F	Lumbar vertebral column myelogram

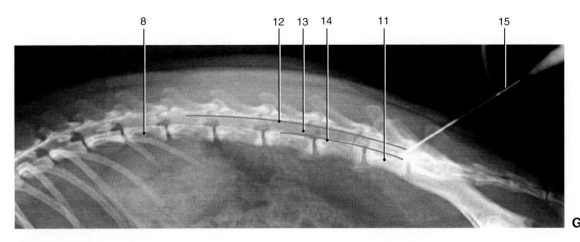

G

Figure 6-23, A-G—cont'd

Type of animal: Guinea pig

Type of study: Myelogram

Contrast medium: Isovue 200 (iopamidol injection 41%, 20% bound iodine; Bracco Diagnostics, Inc., Princeton, NJ); injection site L6-S1

Projection: Laterolateral (right lateral recumbency)

Weight of animal: 1.2 kg

Gender: Male

Reproductive status: Intact

Age: Adult

Image	Projection
G	Lumbar vertebral column test injection

1. Atlas
2. Cervical intervertebral space
3. 7th cervical vertebra
4. 1st thoracic vertebra
5. Thoracic intervertebral space
6. Thoracic intervertebral foramen
7. 13th thoracic vertebra
8. 1st lumbar vertebra
9. Lumbar intervertebral space
10. Lumbar intervertebral foramen
11. 6th lumbar vertebra
12. Dorsal aspect of subarachnoid space
13. Spinal cord
14. Ventral aspect of subarachnoid space
15. Spinal needle

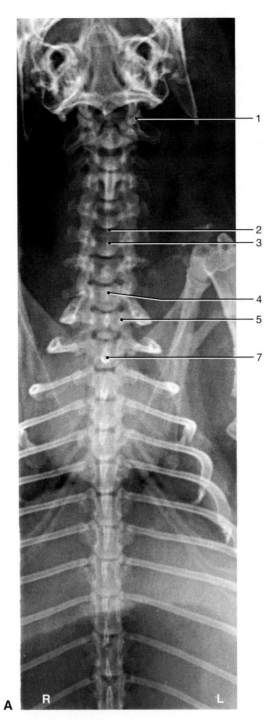

A

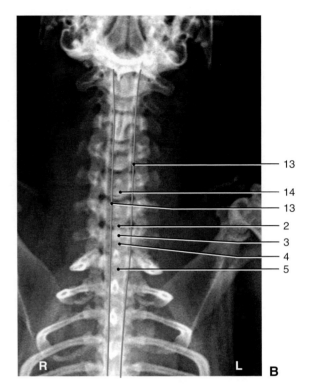

B

1. Atlas
2. Cervical intervertebral space
3. Spinous process of cervical vertebra
4. 7th cervical vertebra
5. 1st thoracic vertebra
6. Thoracic intervertebral space
7. Spinous process of thoracic vertebra
8. 13th thoracic vertebra
9. 1st lumbar vertebra
10. Lumbar intervertebral space
11. Spinous process of lumbar vertebra
12. 6th lumbar vertebra
13. Lateral aspect of subarachnoid space
14. Spinal cord
15. Sacrum

Figure 6-24, A-F
Type of animal: Guinea pig
Type of study: Myelogram
Contrast medium: Isovue 200 (iopamidol injection
    41%, 20% bound iodine; Bracco Diagnostics, Inc.,
    Princeton, NJ); injection site L6-S1
Projection: Dorsoventral
Weight of animal: 1.2 kg
Gender: Male
Reproductive status: Intact
Age: Adult

Image	Projection
A	Cervico-thoracic vertebral column survey
B	Cervical vertebral column myelogram

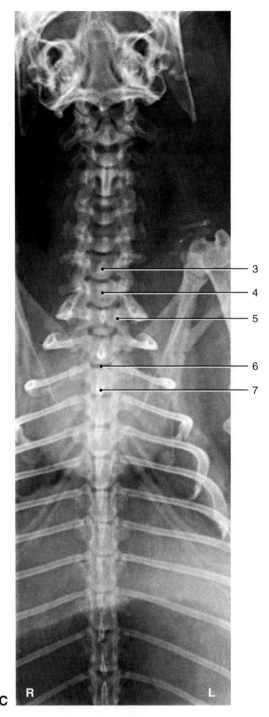

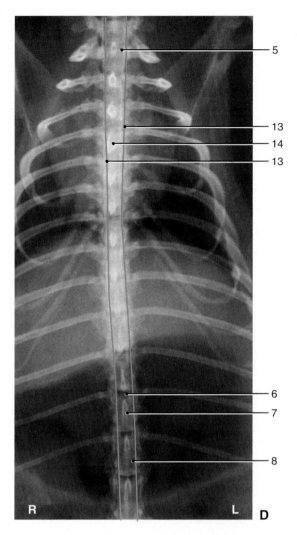

Figure 6-24, A-F—cont'd
Type of animal: Guinea pig
Type of study: Myelogram
Contrast medium: Isovue 200 (iopamidol injection 41%, 20% bound iodine; Bracco Diagnostics, Inc., Princeton, NJ); injection site L6-S1
Projection: Dorsoventral
Weight of animal: 1.2 kg
Gender: Male
Reproductive status: Intact
Age: Adult

1. Atlas
2. Cervical intervertebral space
3. Spinous process of cervical vertebra
4. 7th cervical vertebra
5. 1st thoracic vertebra
6. Thoracic intervertebral space
7. Spinous process of thoracic vertebra
8. 13th thoracic vertebra
9. 1st lumbar vertebra
10. Lumbar intervertebral space
11. Spinous process of lumbar vertebra
12. 6th lumbar vertebra
13. Lateral aspect of subarachnoid space
14. Spinal cord
15. Sacrum

Image	Projection
C	Cervico-thoracic column survey
D	Thoracic vertebral column myelogram

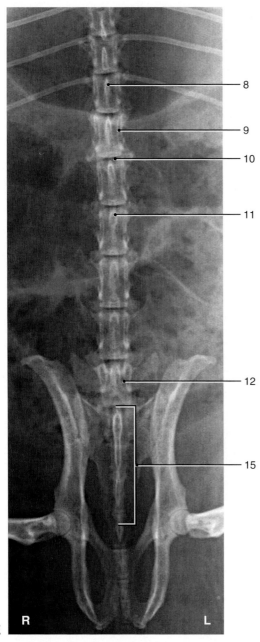

E

Figure 6-24, A-F—cont'd
Type of animal: Guinea pig
Type of study: Myelogram
Contrast medium: Isovue 200 (iopamidol injection
    41%, 20% bound iodine; Bracco Diagnostics, Inc.,
    Princeton, NJ); injection site L6-S1
Projection: Dorsoventral
Weight of animal: 1.2 kg
Gender: Male
Reproductive status: Intact
Age: Adult

Image	Projection
E	Lumbar vertebral column survey
F	Lumbar vertebral column myelogram

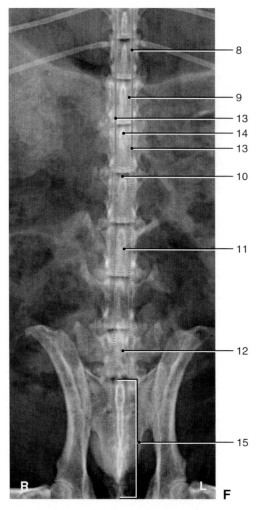

F

1. Atlas
2. Cervical intervertebral space
3. Spinous process of cervical vertebra
4. 7th cervical vertebra
5. 1st thoracic vertebra
6. Thoracic intervertebral space
7. Spinous process of thoracic vertebra
8. 13th thoracic vertebra
9. 1st lumbar vertebra
10. Lumbar intervertebral space
11. Spinous process of lumbar vertebra
12. 6th lumbar vertebra
13. Lateral aspect of subarachnoid space
14. Spinal cord
15. Sacrum

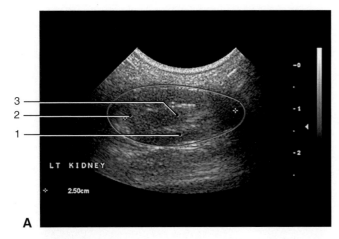

Figure 6-25, A
Sagittal image of left kidney

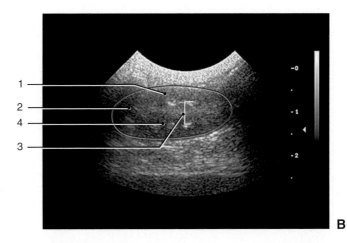

Figure 6-25, B
Sagittal image of left kidney

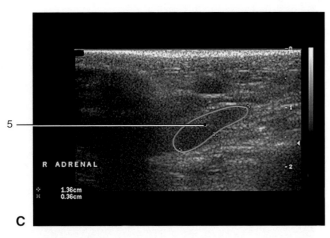

Figure 6-25, C
Sagittal image of right adrenal gland

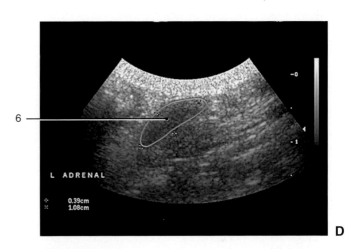

Figure 6-25, D
Sagittal image of left adrenal gland

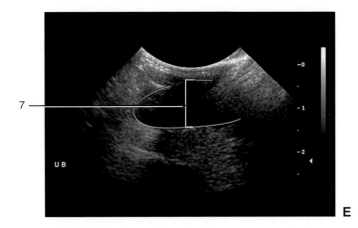

Figure 6-25, E
Sagittal image of urinary bladder

Figure 6-25, A-E
Type of animal: Guinea pig
Type of study: Ultrasound study of urinary tract
    and associated structures
Weight of animal: 1 kg
Gender: Female
Reproductive status: Intact
Age: 1 year

1. Renal cortex
2. Cranial pole of kidney
3. Renal pelvis
4. Renal medulla
5. Right adrenal gland
6. Left adrenal gland
7. Urinary bladder

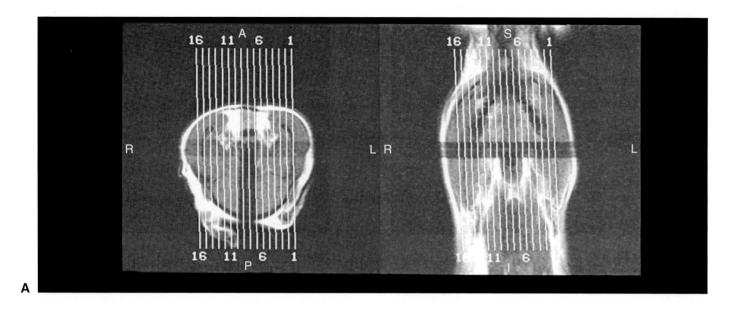

A

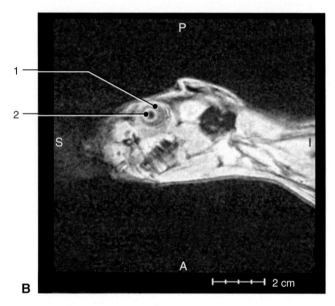

B

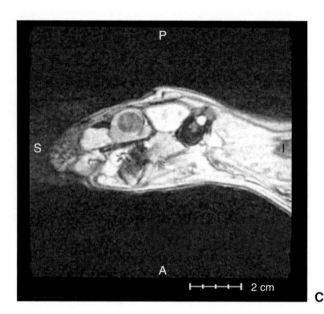

C

Figure 6-26, A-F
Type of Animal: Guinea pig
Type of Study: MRI head
Image Plane: Sagittal

1. Eyeball
2. Lens of eyeball
3. Nasal cavity
4. Cerebellum
5. Cerebrum
6. Olfactory bulb
7. Nasoturbinates
8. Mandible
9. Trachea
10. Spinal cord
11. Nasopharynx
12. Tongue
13. Brain stem

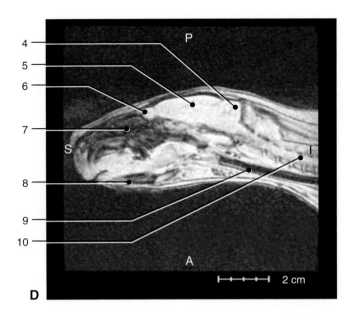

D

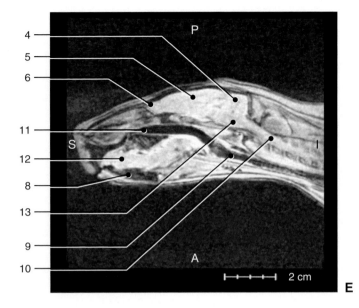

E

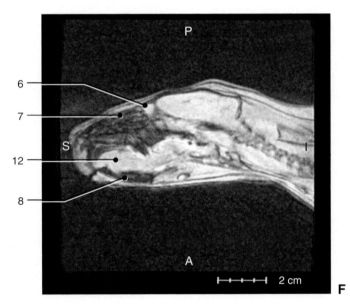

F

Figure 6-26, A-F—cont'd
Type of Animal: Guinea pig
Type of Study: MRI head
Image Plane: Sagittal

1. Eyeball
2. Lens of eyeball
3. Nasal cavity
4. Cerebellum
5. Cerebrum
6. Olfactory bulb
7. Nasoturbinates
8. Mandible
9. Trachea
10. Spinal cord
11. Nasopharynx
12. Tongue
13. Brain stem

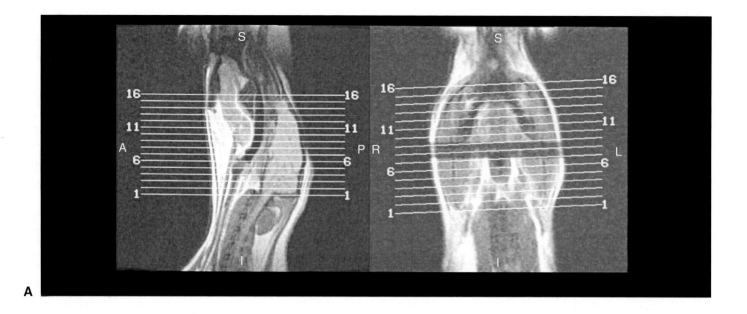

A

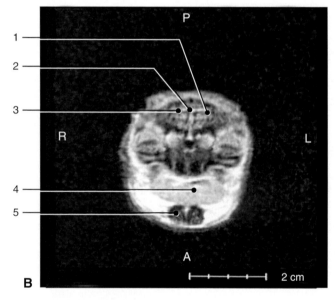

B

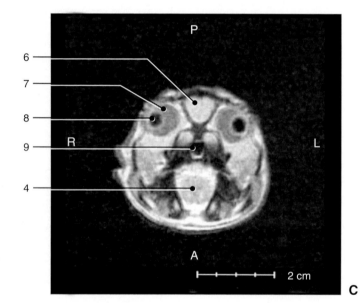

C

Figure 6-27, A-G
Type of animal: Guinea pig
Type of study: MRI head
Imaging plane: Transverse

1. Nasal cavity
2. Nasal septum
3. Nasoturbinates
4. Tongue
5. Mandible
6. Olfactory bulb
7. Eyeball
8. Lens of eyeball
9. Nasopharynx
10. Cerebrum
11. Masseter muscle
12. Cerebral aqueduct
13. Tympanic cavity
14. Larynx
15. Cerebellum
16. Brain stem
17. Trachea

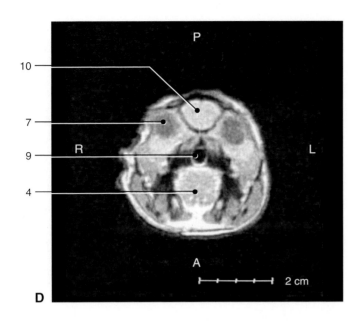

D

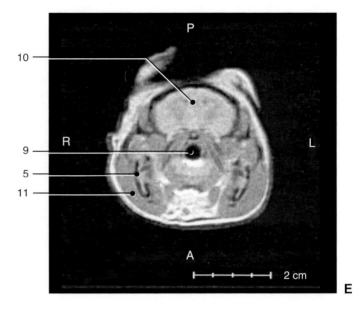

E

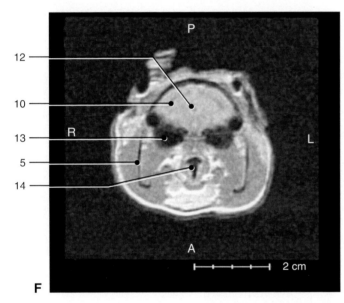

F

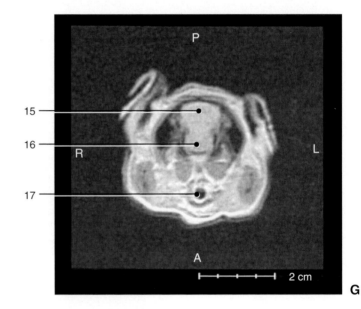

G

Figure 6-27, A-G—cont'd
Type of animal: Guinea pig
Type of study: MRI head
Imaging plane: Transverse

1. Nasal cavity
2. Nasal septum
3. Nasoturbinates
4. Tongue
5. Mandible
6. Olfactory bulb
7. Eyeball
8. Lens of eyeball
9. Nasopharynx
10. Cerebrum
11. Masseter muscle
12. Cerebral aqueduct
13. Tympanic cavity
14. Larynx
15. Cerebellum
16. Brain stem
17. Trachea

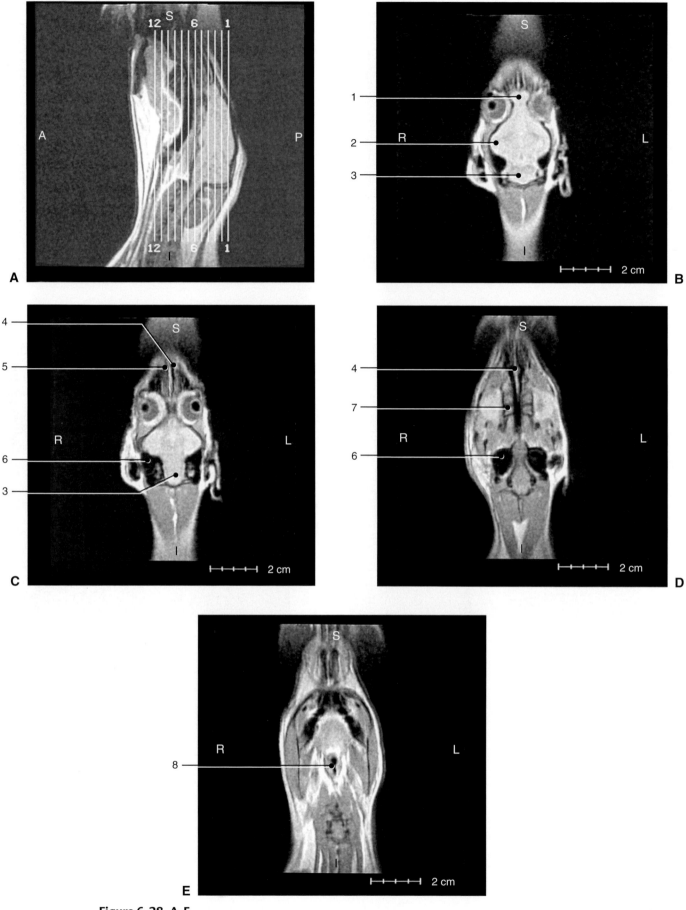

Figure 6-28, A-E

Type of animal: Guinea pig

Type of study: MRI head

Imaging plane: Coronal

1. Olfactory bulb
2. Cerebrum
3. Cerebellum
4. Nasal septum
5. Nasal cavity
6. Tympanic cavity
7. Molar teeth
8. Larynx

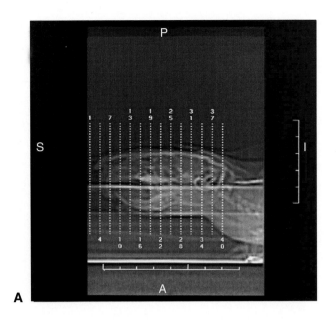

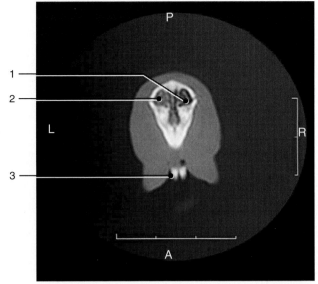

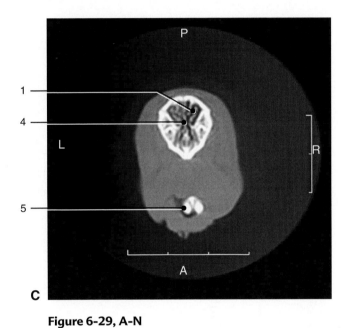

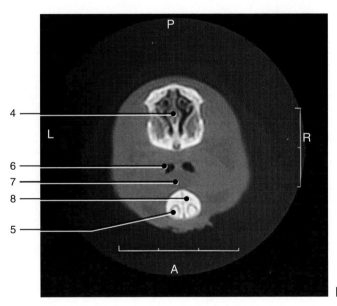

Figure 6-29, A-N

Type of animal: Guinea pig
Type of study: CT head
Imaging plane: Transverse
Weight of animal: 1.2 kg
Gender: Male
Reproductive status: Intact
Age: 1.5 years

1. Nasoturbinates
2. Nasal cavity
3. Maxillary incisor tooth
4. Nasal septum
5. Mandibular incisor tooth
6. Oral cavity
7. Tongue
8. Mandible
9. Ethmoturbinates
10. Molar tooth
11. Zygomatic process of maxilla
12. Cribriform plate
13. Eyeball
14. Zygomatic bone
15. Cerebrum

16. Nasopharynx
17. Basisphenoidal bone
18. Pterygoid muscle
19. Temporomandibular joint
20. Mandible
21. Hyoid bone
22. Tympanic cavity
23. Tympanic bulla
24. Occipital bone
25. Larynx
26. Ear canal (calcified)
27. Ear canal
28. Occipital condyle
29. Dorsal sagittal crest
30. Atlas

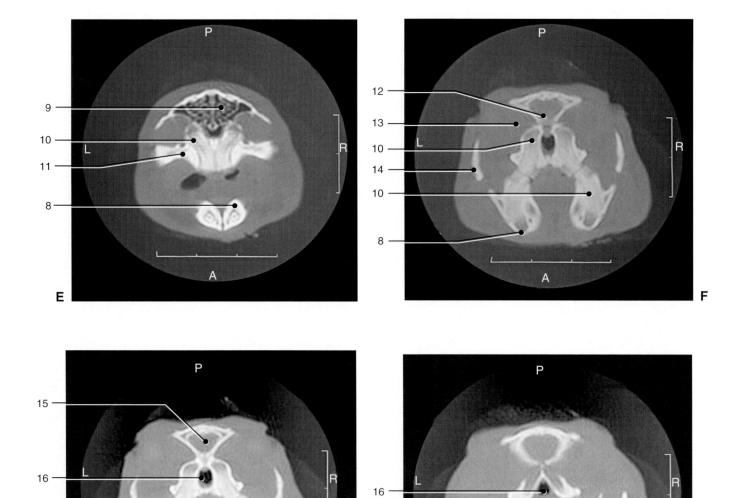

Figure 6-29, A-N—cont'd
Type of animal: Guinea pig
Type of study: CT head
Imaging plane: Transverse
Weight of animal: 1.2 kg
Gender: Male
Reproductive status: Intact
Age: 1.5 years

1. Nasoturbinates
2. Nasal cavity
3. Maxillary incisor tooth
4. Nasal septum
5. Mandibular incisor tooth
6. Oral cavity
7. Tongue
8. Mandible
9. Ethmoturbinates
10. Molar tooth
11. Zygomatic process of maxilla
12. Cribriform plate
13. Eyeball
14. Zygomatic bone
15. Cerebrum

16. Nasopharynx
17. Basisphenoidal bone
18. Pterygoid muscle
19. Temporomandibular joint
20. Mandible
21. Hyoid bone
22. Tympanic cavity
23. Tympanic bulla
24. Occipital bone
25. Larynx
26. Ear canal (calcified)
27. Ear canal
28. Occipital condyle
29. Dorsal sagittal crest
30. Atlas

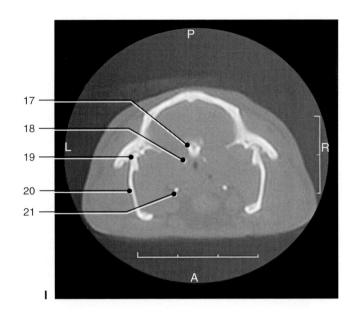

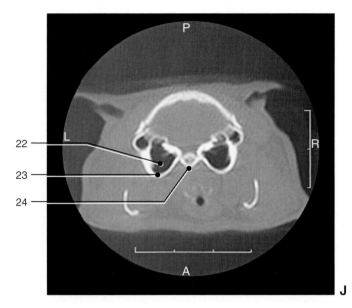

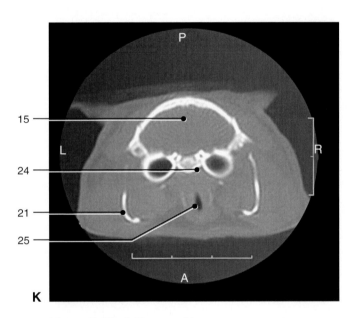

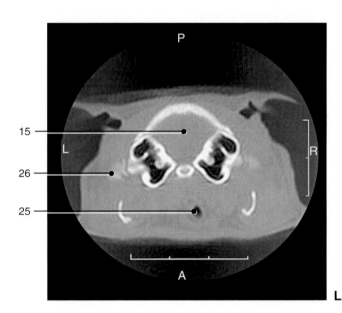

Figure 6-29, A-N—cont'd
Type of animal: Guinea pig
Type of study: CT head
Imaging plane: Transverse
Weight of animal: 1.2 kg
Gender: Male
Reproductive status: Intact
Age: 1.5 years

1. Nasoturbinates
2. Nasal cavity
3. Maxillary incisor tooth
4. Nasal septum
5. Mandibular incisor tooth
6. Oral cavity
7. Tongue
8. Mandible
9. Ethmoturbinates
10. Molar tooth
11. Zygomatic process of maxilla
12. Cribriform plate
13. Eyeball
14. Zygomatic bone
15. Cerebrum

16. Nasopharynx
17. Basisphenoidal bone
18. Pterygoid muscle
19. Temporomandibular joint
20. Mandible
21. Hyoid bone
22. Tympanic cavity
23. Tympanic bulla
24. Occipital bone
25. Larynx
26. Ear canal (calcified)
27. Ear canal
28. Occipital condyle
29. Dorsal sagittal crest
30. Atlas

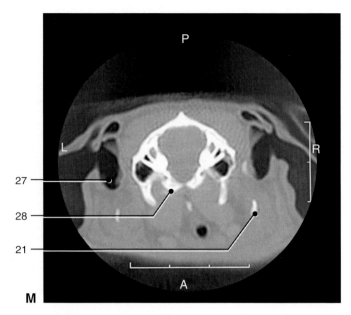

M

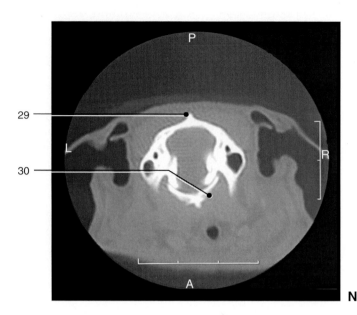

N

Figure 6-29, A-N—cont'd
Type of animal: Guinea pig
Type of study: CT head
Imaging plane: Transverse
Weight of animal: 1.2 kg
Gender: Male
Reproductive status: Intact
Age: 1.5 years

1. Nasoturbinates
2. Nasal cavity
3. Maxillary incisor tooth
4. Nasal septum
5. Mandibular incisor tooth
6. Oral cavity
7. Tongue
8. Mandible
9. Ethmoturbinates
10. Molar tooth
11. Zygomatic process of maxilla
12. Cribriform plate
13. Eyeball
14. Zygomatic bone
15. Cerebrum

16. Nasopharynx
17. Basisphenoidal bone
18. Pterygoid muscle
19. Temporomandibular joint
20. Mandible
21. Hyoid bone
22. Tympanic cavity
23. Tympanic bulla
24. Occipital bone
25. Larynx
26. Ear canal (calcified)
27. Ear canal
28. Occipital condyle
29. Dorsal sagittal crest
30. Atlas

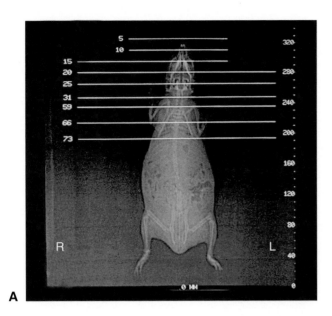

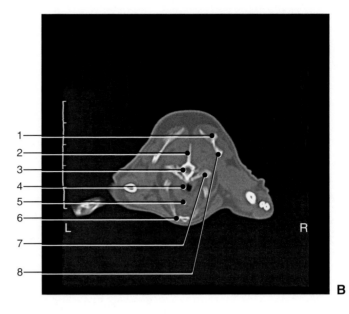

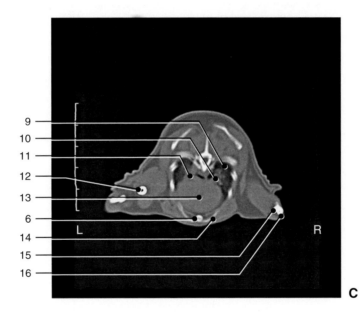

Figure 6-30, A-E
Type of animal: Guinea pig
Type of study: CT thorax
Imaging plane: Transverse

1. Spine of scapula
2. Spinous process of thoracic vertebra
3. Spinal canal of thoracic vertebra
4. Trachea
5. Cranial mediastinum
6. Sternebra
7. Rib
8. Scapula
9. Lung
10. Pulmonary artery
11. Aorta

12. Humerus
13. Heart
14. Costal cartilage
15. Ulna
16. Radius
17. Bronchus
18. Pulmonary vein
19. Elbow joint
20. Caudal vena cava
21. Liver

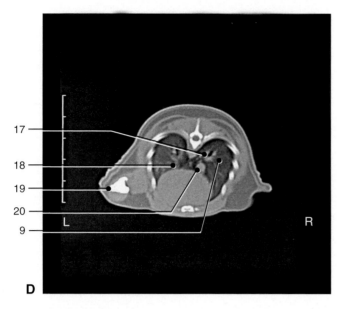

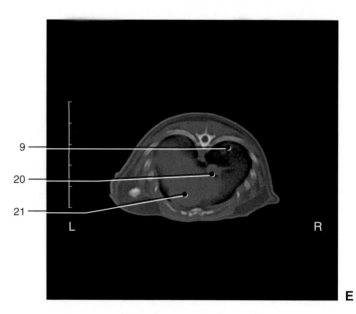

Figure 6-30, A-E
Type of animal: Guinea pig
Type of study: CT thorax
Imaging plane: Transverse

1. Spine of scapula
2. Spinous process of thoracic vertebra
3. Spinal canal of thoracic vertebra
4. Trachea
5. Cranial mediastinum
6. Sternebra
7. Rib
8. Scapula
9. Lung
10. Pulmonary artery
11. Aorta

12. Humerus
13. Heart
14. Costal cartilage
15. Ulna
16. Radius
17. Bronchus
18. Pulmonary vein
19. Elbow joint
20. Caudal vena cava
21. Liver

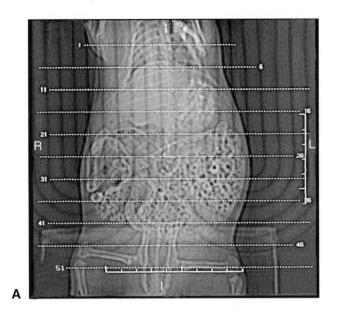

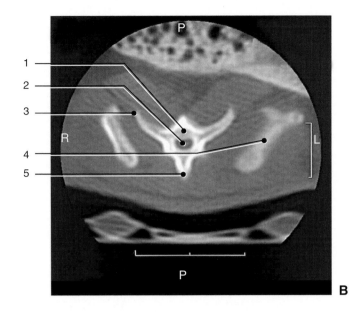

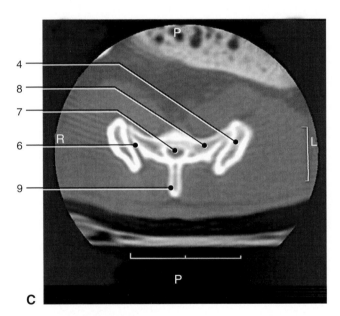

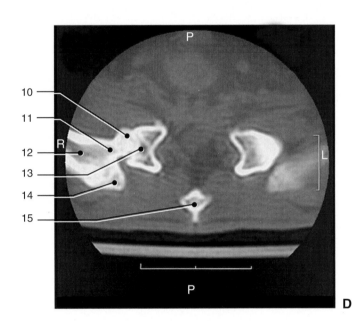

Figure 6-31, A-D

Type of animal: Guinea pig
Type of study: CT pelvis
Imaging plane: Transverse
Weight of animal: 1.2 kg
Gender: Male
Reproductive status: Intact
Age: Adult

1. Lumbar vertebra
2. Spinal canal of lumbar vertebra
3. Transverse process of lumbar vertebra
4. Ilium
5. Spinous process of lumbar vertebra
6. Sacroiliac joint
7. Spinal canal of sacral vertebra
8. Sacral vertebra

9. Spinous process of sacral vertebra
10. Femoral head
11. Femoral neck
12. Femur
13. Acetabulum
14. Greater trochanter of femur
15. Caudal vertebra

CHAPTER • 7

Domestic Rabbit *(Oryctolagus cuniculus)*

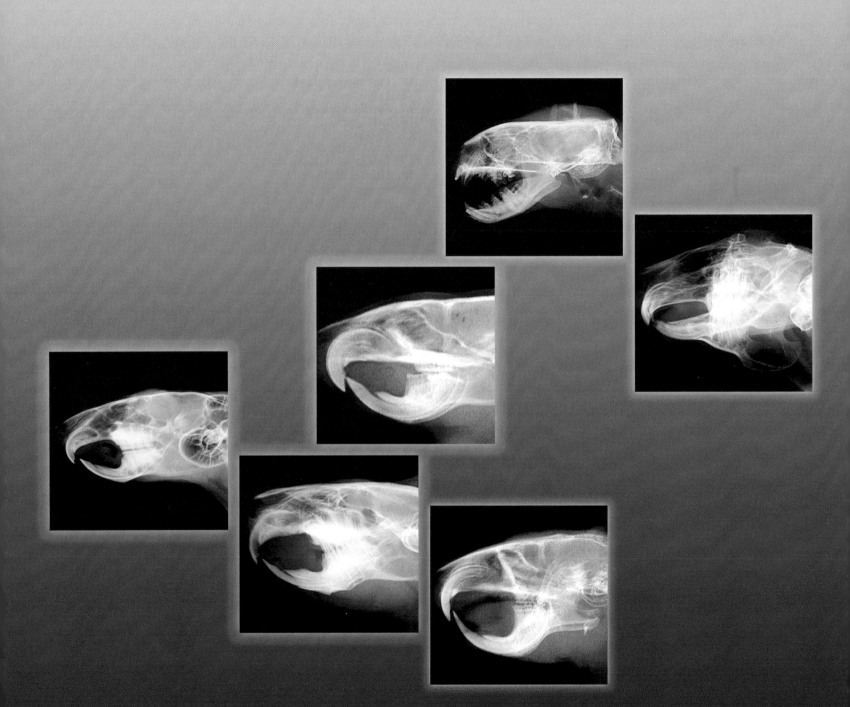

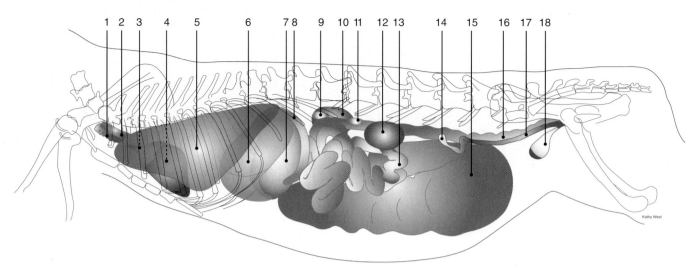

Figure 7-1, A Anatomic drawing (view of the left side) of viscera of the thorax and abdomen of an adult female rabbit.

1. Trachea
2. Esophagus
3. Thymus
4. Heart
5. Lung
6. Liver
7. Stomach
8. Spleen
9. Right adrenal gland
10. Right kidney
11. Left adrenal gland
12. Left kidney
13. Small intestine
14. Left ovary
15. Cecum
16. Descending colon
17. Left horn of uterus
18. Urinary bladder

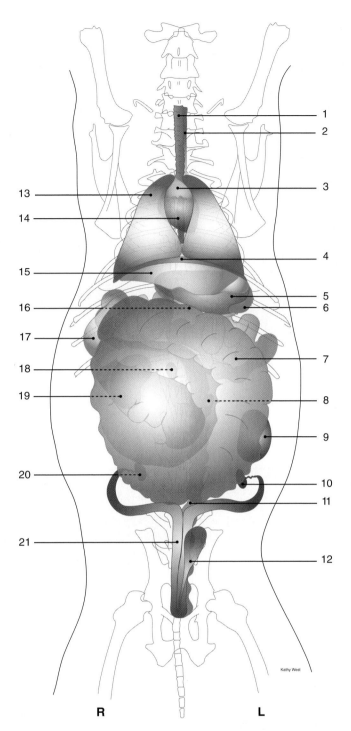

Figure 7-1, B Anatomic drawing (ventrodorsal view) of viscera of the thorax and abdomen of an adult female rabbit.

1. Trachea
2. Esophagus
3. Thymus
4. Diaphragm
5. Stomach
6. Spleen
7. Cecum
8. Left adrenal gland
9. Left kidney
10. Left ovary
11. Descending colon
12. Urinary bladder
13. Lung
14. Heart
15. Liver
16. Pancreas
17. Small intestine
18. Right adrenal gland
19. Right kidney
20. Right ovary
21. Right horn of uterus

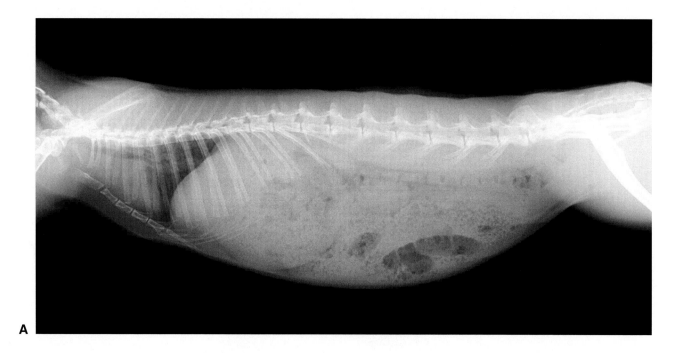

A

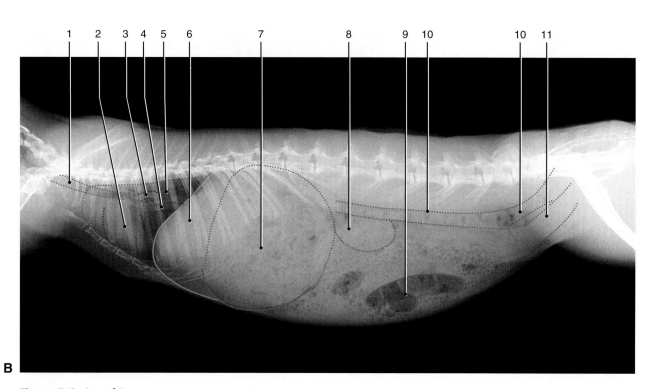

B

Figure 7-2, A and B
Type of animal: Rabbit
Type of study: Viscera of thorax and abdomen
Projection: Laterolateral (right lateral recumbency)
Weight of animal: 2.2 kg
Gender: Male
Reproductive status: Neutered
Age: Adult

1. Trachea
2. Heart
3. Pulmonary vasculature
4. Caudal vena cava
5. Lung
6. Liver

7. Stomach
8. Kidney
9. Cecum
10. Colon
11. Urinary bladder

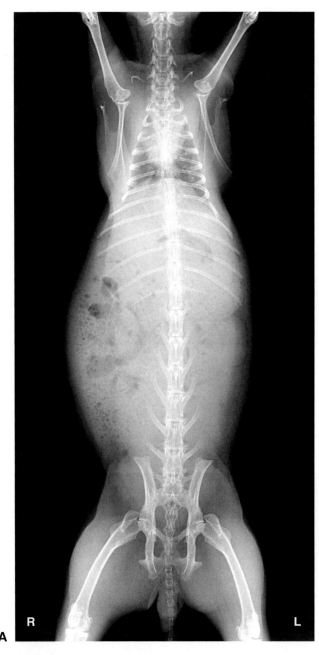

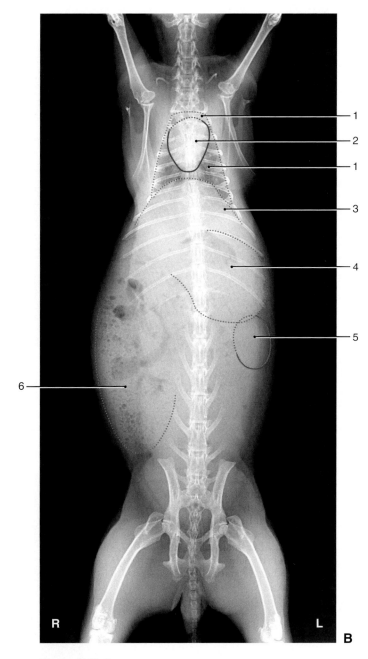

Figure 7-3, A
Type of animal: Rabbit
Type of study: Viscera of thorax and abdomen
Projection: Ventrodorsal
Weight of animal: 2.2 kg
Gender: Male
Reproductive status: Neutered
Age: Adult

Figure 7-3, B
Type of animal: Rabbit
Type of study: Viscera of thorax and abdomen
Projection: Ventrodorsal
Weight of animal: 2.2 kg
Gender: Male
Reproductive status: Neutered
Age: Adult

1. Lung
2. Heart
3. Liver
4. Stomach
5. Left kidney
6. Cecum

Figure 7-4, A
Type of animal: Rabbit
Type of study: Head
Projection: Laterolateral
　(right lateral recumbency)
Weight of animal: 4.1 kg
Gender: Female
Reproductive status: Intact
Age: Adult

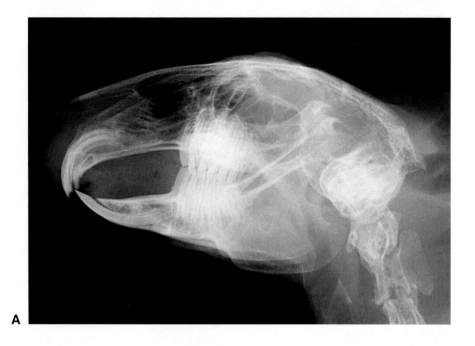

A

Figure 7-4, B
Type of animal: Rabbit
Type of study: Head
Projection: Laterolateral
　(right lateral recumbency)
Weight of animal: 4.1 kg
Gender: Female
Reproductive status: Intact
Age: Adult

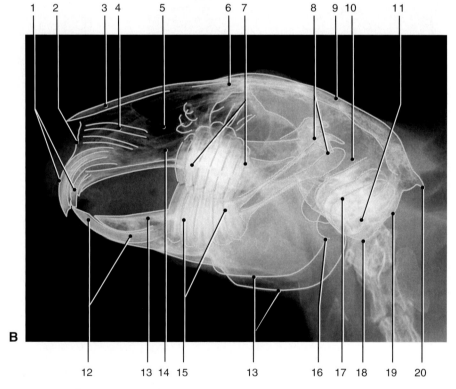

B

1. Maxillary incisor teeth
2. Incisive bone
3. Nasal bone
4. Nasoturbinates
5. Nasal cavity
6. Frontal bone
7. Maxillary premolar and
　molar teeth
8. Condylar processes of mandible
9. Parietal bone
10. Temporal bone
11. Tympanic cavity
12. Mandibular incisor tooth
13. Mandible
14. Maxilla
15. Mandibular premolar and
　molar teeth
16. Angular process of mandible
17. Tympanic bulla
18. Occipital condyle
19. Occipital bone
20. External occipital protuberance

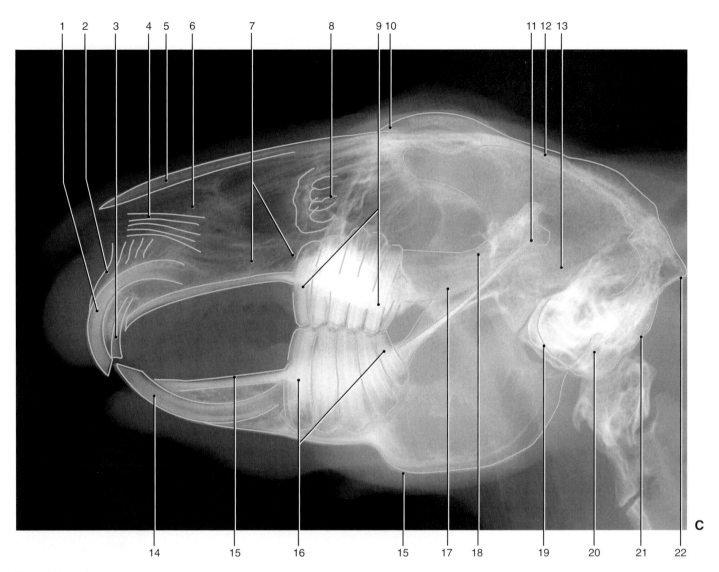

Figure 7-4, C
Type of animal: Rabbit
Type of study: Magnification study of head
Projection: Laterolateral (right lateral recumbency)

1. Maxillary incisor tooth
2. Incisive bone
3. 2nd maxillary incisor tooth
4. Nasoturbinates
5. Nasal bone
6. Nasal cavity
7. Maxilla
8. Ethmoturbinates
9. Maxillary premolar and molar teeth
10. Frontal bone
11. Condylar process of mandible

12. Parietal bone
13. Temporal bone
14. Mandibular incisor tooth
15. Mandible
16. Mandibular premolar and molar teeth
17. Rostral margin of mandibular ramus
18. Zygomatic bone
19. Tympanic bulla
20. Tympanic cavity
21. Occipital bone
22. External occipital protuberance

Figure 7-5, A
Type of animal: Rabbit
Type of study: Head
Projection: Oblique
(30 degree) ventrodorsal
Weight of animal: 4.1 kg
Gender: Female
Reproductive status: Intact
Age: Adult

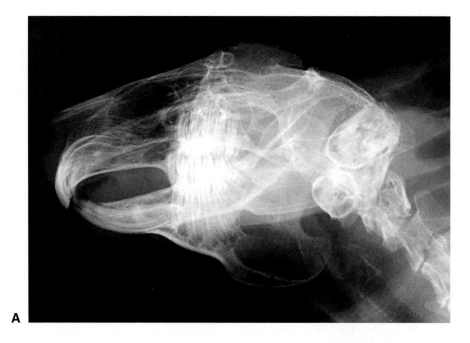

A

Figure 7-5, B
Type of animal: Rabbit
Type of study: Head
Projection: Oblique
(30 degree) ventrodorsal
Weight of animal: 4.1 kg
Gender: Female
Reproductive status: Intact
Age: Adult

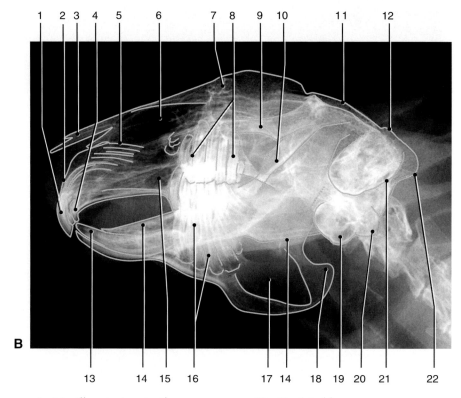

B

1. Maxillary incisor tooth
2. Incisive bone
3. Nasal bone
4. 2nd maxillary incisor tooth
5. Nasoturbinates
6. Nasal cavity
7. Frontal bone
8. Maxillary premolar and molar teeth
9. Zygomatic bone
10. Rostral margin of mandible
11. Parietal bone
12. Occipital bone
13. Mandibular incisor tooth
14. Mandible
15. Maxilla
16. Mandibular premolar and molar teeth
17. Masseteric fossa of mandible
18. Angular process of mandible
19. Tympanic cavity
20. Occipital condyle
21. Tympanic bulla
22. External occipital protuberance

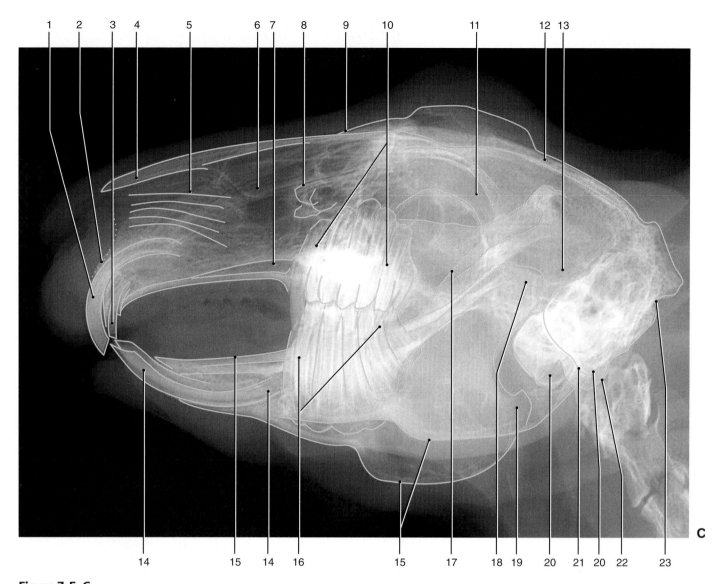

Figure 7-5, C
Type of animal: Rabbit
Type of study: Magnification study of head
Projection: Oblique (10 degree) ventrodorsal

1. Maxillary incisor tooth
2. Incisive bone
3. 2nd maxillary incisor tooth
4. Nasal bone
5. Nasoturbinates
6. Nasal cavity
7. Maxilla
8. Ethmoturbinates
9. Frontal bone
10. Maxillary premolar and molar teeth
11. Zygomatic bone
12. Parietal bone
13. Temporal bone
14. Mandibular incisor tooth
15. Mandible
16. Mandibular premolar and molar teeth
17. Coronoid process of mandible
18. Condylar process of mandible
19. Angular process of mandible
20. Tympanic cavity
21. Tympanic bulla
22. Occipital condyle
23. Occipital bone

Figure 7-6, A
Type of animal: Rabbit
Type of study: Head
Projection: Dorsoventral
Weight of animal: 4.1 kg
Gender: Female
Reproductive status: Intact
Age: Adult

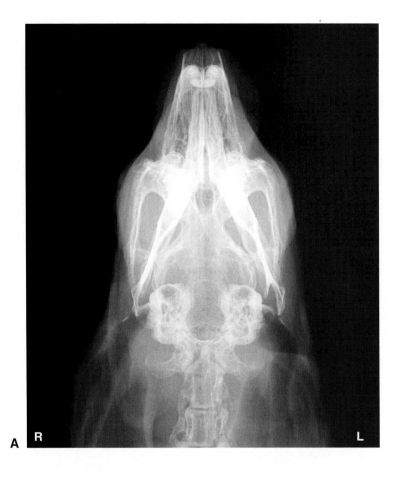

Figure 7-6, B
Type of animal: Rabbit
Type of study: Head
Projection: Dorsoventral
Weight of animal: 4.1 kg
Gender: Female
Reproductive status: Intact
Age: Adult

1. Nasal bone
2. Maxillary incisor tooth
3. 2nd maxillary incisor tooth
4. Incisive bone
5. Maxilla
6. Zygomatic process of maxilla
7. Zygomatic bone
8. Angular process of mandible
9. Tympanic cavity
10. Tympanic bulla
11. Foramen magnum
12. Mandibular incisor tooth
13. 1st maxillary premolar
14. Facial tuber of maxilla
15. Palatine bone
16. Mandible
17. Pterygoid bone
18. Basisphenoidal bone
19. Ear canal
20. Occipital bone

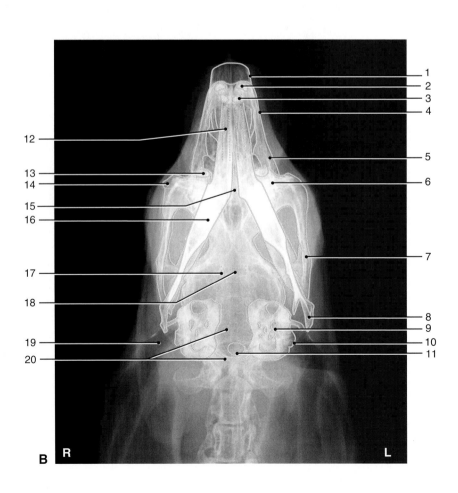

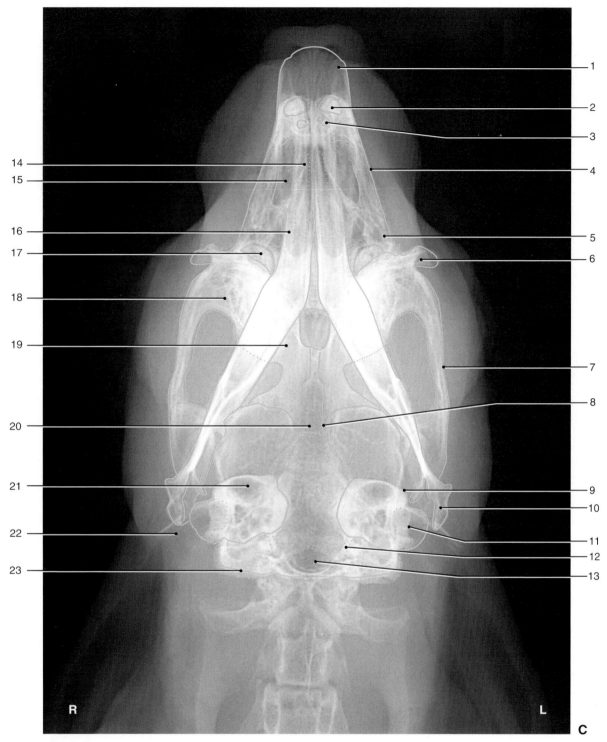

Figure 7-6, C
Type of animal: Rabbit
Type of study: Magnification study of head
Projection: Dorsoventral

1. Nasal bone
2. Maxillary incisor tooth
3. 2nd maxillary incisor tooth
4. Incisive bone
5. Maxilla
6. Facial tuber of maxilla
7. Zygomatic bone
8. Pterygoid bone
9. Tympanic bulla
10. Angular process of mandible
11. External acoustic meatus
12. Occipital condyle
13. Foramen magnum
14. Mandibular incisor tooth
15. Nasal cavity
16. Mandible
17. 1st maxillary premolar tooth
18. Zygomatic process of maxilla
19. Palatine bone
20. Basisphenoidal bone
21. Tympanic cavity
22. Ear canal
23. Occipital bone

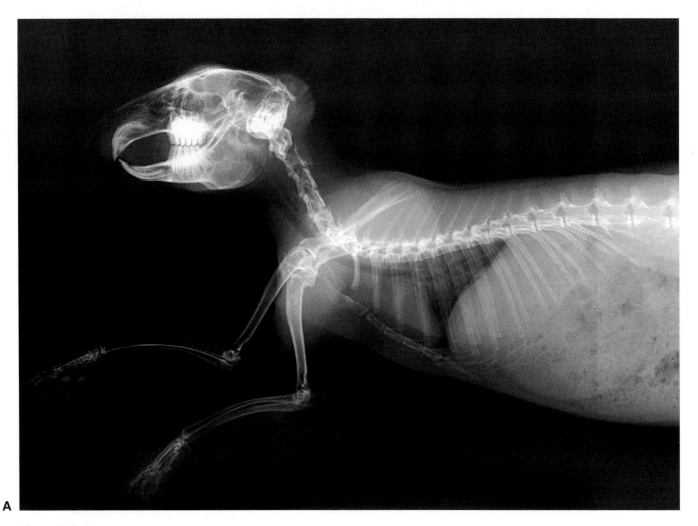

Figure 7-7, A
Type of animal: Rabbit
Type of study: Cervical and thoracic vertebral column
Projection: Laterolateral (right lateral recumbency)
Weight of animal: 2.2 kg
Gender: Male
Reproductive status: Neutered
Age: Adult

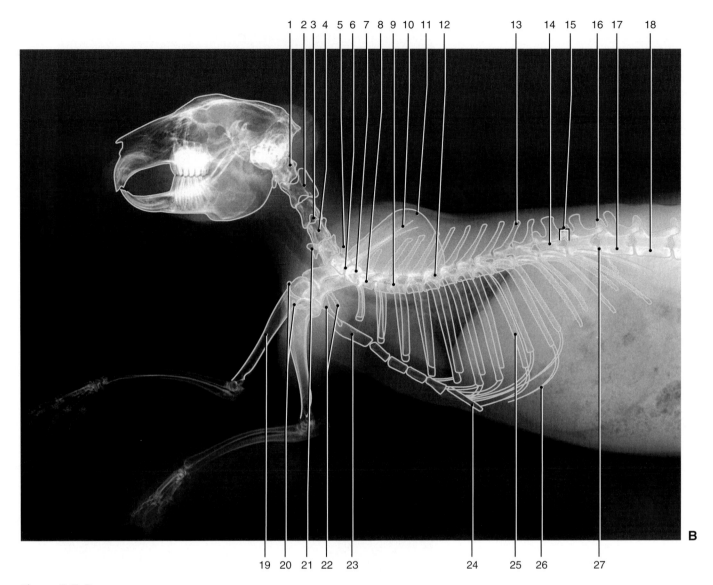

Figure 7-7, B
Type of animal: Rabbit
Type of study: Cervical and thoracic vertebral column
Projection: Laterolateral (right lateral recumbency)
Weight of animal: 2.2 kg
Gender: Male
Reproductive status: Neutered
Age: Adult

1. Atlas
2. Spinous process of axis
3. Cervical intervertebral foramen
4. Cervical spinal canal
5. Spinous process of cervical vertebra
6. Cervical intervertebral space
7. 7th cervical vertebra
8. 1st thoracic vertebra
9. Head of rib
10. Spine of scapula
11. Scapula
12. Thoracic intervertebral foramen
13. Spinous process of thoracic vertebra
14. Thoracic spinal canal
15. Articular processes of thoracic vertebrae
16. Mammillary process of thoracic vertebra
17. 13th thoracic vertebra
18. 1st lumbar vertebra
19. Humerus
20. Clavicles
21. Transverse process of cervical vertebra
22. Suprahamate processes
23. Manubrium of sternum
24. Xyphoid process
25. Rib
26. Costal cartilage
27. Thoracic intervertebral space

Figure 7-8, A
Type of animal: Rabbit
Type of study: Cervical and thoracic
  vertebral column
Projection: Ventrodorsal
Weight of animal: 2.2 kg
Gender: Male
Reproductive status: Neutered
Age: Adult

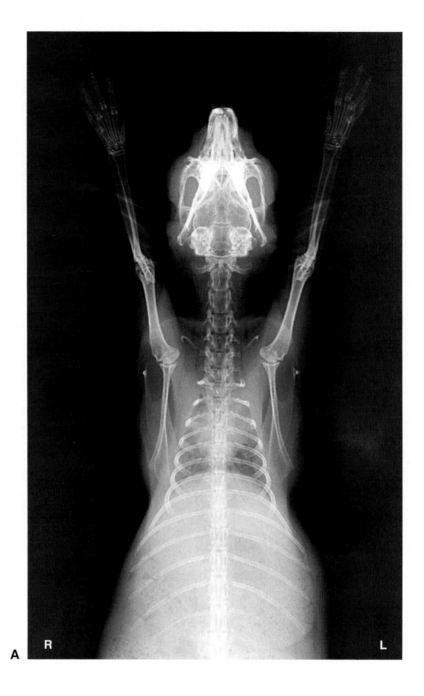

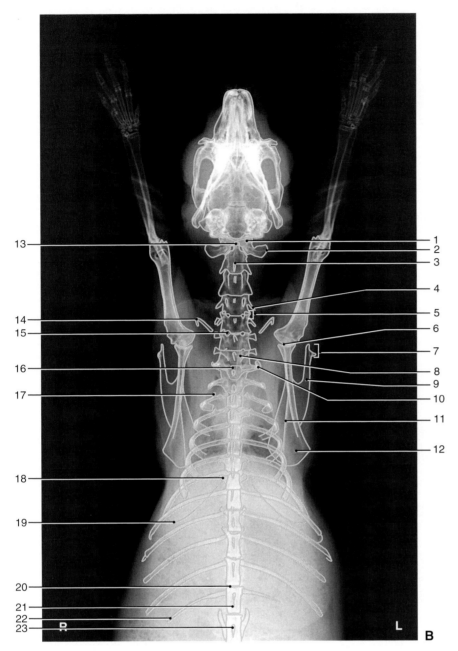

Figure 7-8, B
Type of animal: Rabbit
Type of study: Cervical and
    thoracic vertebral column
Projection: Ventrodorsal
Weight of animal: 2.2 kg
Gender: Male
Reproductive status: Neutered
Age: Adult

1. Atlas
2. Transverse process of atlas
3. Spinous process of axis
4. Transverse process of cervical
   vertebra
5. Articular processes of cervical
   vertebrae
6. Scapulohumeral joint space
7. Suprahamate process
8. 7th cervical vertebra
9. Acromion
10. 1st rib
11. Spine of scapula
12. Scapula
13. Dens of axis
14. Clavicle
15. Cervical intervertebral space
16. 1st thoracic vertebra
17. Tubercle of rib
18. Transverse process of thoracic
    vertebra
19. Costal cartilage
20. Thoracic intervertebral space
21. 13th thoracic vertebra
22. 13th rib
23. 1st lumbar vertebra

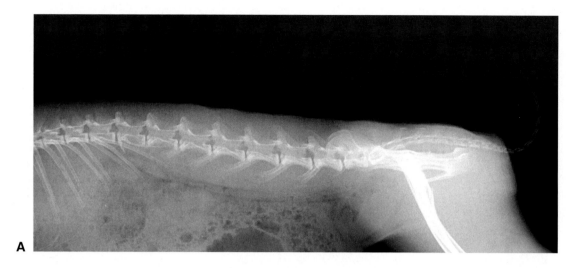

A

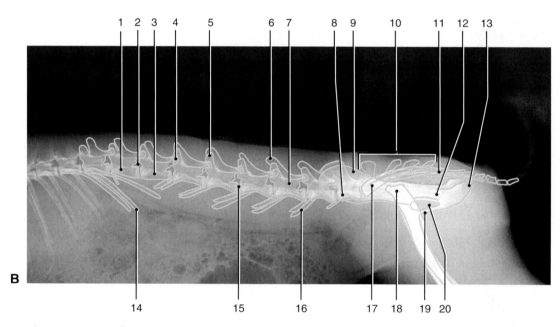

B

Figure 7-9, A and B
Type of animal: Rabbit
Type of study: Lumbar, sacral, and caudal vertebral column
Projection: Laterolateral (right lateral recumbency)
Weight of animal: 2.2 kg
Gender: Male
Reproductive status: Neutered
Age: Adult

1. 13th thoracic vertebra
2. Thoracolumbar intervertebral foramen
3. 1st lumbar vertebra
4. Articular processes of lumbar vertebra
5. Mammillary process of lumbar vertebra
6. Spinous process of lumbar vertebra
7. Spinal canal
8. 7th lumbar vertebra
9. Ilium
10. Spinous processes of sacral vertebrae
11. 1st caudal vertebra
12. Ischium
13. Ischial tuberosity
14. 12th rib
15. Lumbar intervertebral space
16. Transverse process of lumbar vertebra
17. Sacrum
18. Femoral head
19. Pubis
20. Obturator foramen

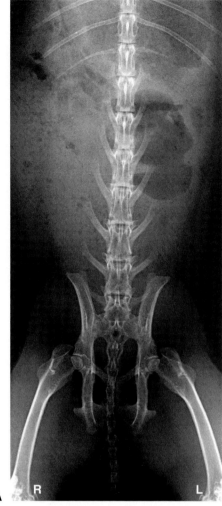

Figure 7-10, A
Type of animal: Rabbit
Type of study: Lumbar, sacral,
  and caudal vertebral column
Projection: Ventrodorsal
Weight of animal: 2.2 kg
Gender: Male
Reproductive status: Neutered
Age: Adult

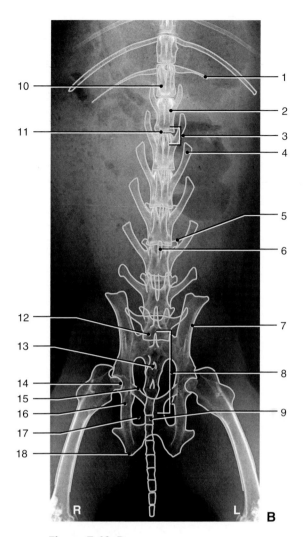

Figure 7-10, B
Type of animal: Rabbit
Type of study: Lumbar, sacral,
  and caudal vertebral column
Projection: Ventrodorsal
Weight of animal: 2.2 kg
Gender: Male
Reproductive status: Neutered
Age: Adult

1. 13th rib
2. 1st lumbar vertebra
3. Articular processes of lumbar vertebrae
4. Transverse process of lumbar vertebra
5. Mammillary process of lumbar vertebra
6. Spinous process of lumbar vertebra
7. Ilium
8. Sacrum
9. 1st caudal vertebra
10. 13th thoracic vertebra
11. Lumbar intervertebral space
12. 7th lumbar vertebra
13. Spinous process of sacral vertebra
14. Acetabulum
15. Pubis
16. Ischium
17. Obturator foramen
18. Ischial tuberosity

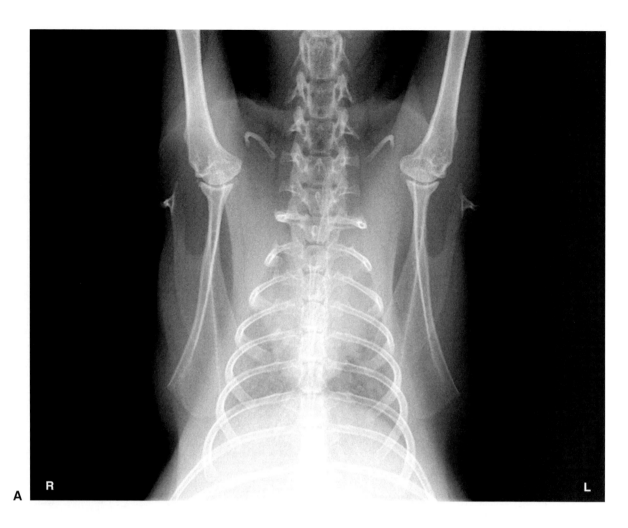

Figure 7-11, A
Type of animal: Rabbit
Type of study: Scapula
Projection: Caudocranial
Weight of animal: 2.2 kg
Gender: Male
Reproductive status: Neutered
Age: Adult

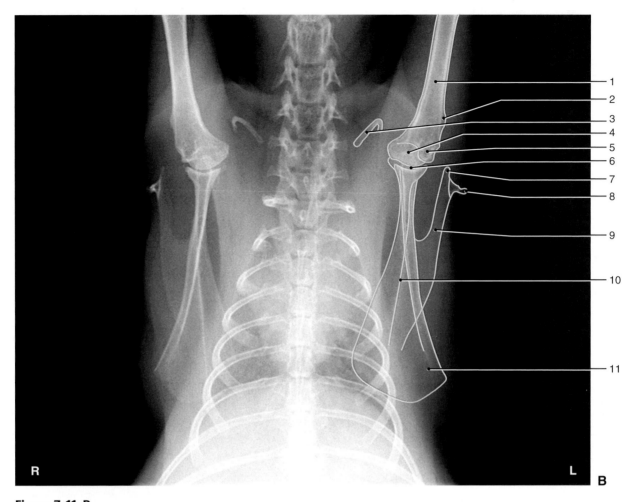

Figure 7-11, B
Type of animal: Rabbit
Type of study: Scapula
Projection: Caudocranial
Weight of animal: 2.2 kg
Gender: Male
Reproductive status: Neutered
Age: Adult

1. Humerus
2. Deltoid tuberosity of humerus
3. Clavicle
4. Humeral head
5. Greater tubercle of humerus
6. Scapulohumeral joint space
7. Hamate process
8. Suprahamate process
9. Acromion
10. Spine of scapula
11. Scapula

Figure 7-12, A
Type of animal: Rabbit
Type of study: Thoracic limb
Projection: Mediolateral
Weight of animal: 2.2 kg
Gender: Male
Reproductive status: Neutered
Age: Adult

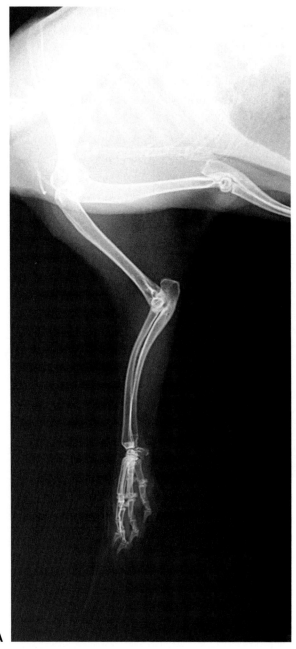

A

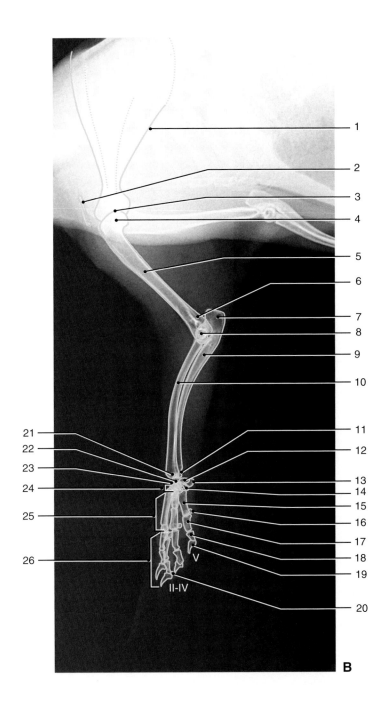

Figure 7-12, B
Type of animal: Rabbit
Type of study: Thoracic limb
Projection: Mediolateral
Weight of animal: 2.2 kg
Gender: Male
Reproductive status: Neutered
Age: Adult

1. Scapula
2. Clavicle
3. Scapulohumeral joint space
4. Humeral head
5. Humerus
6. Humeral epicondyle
7. Olecranon of ulna
8. Humeral condyle
9. Ulna
10. Radius
11. Styloid process of ulna
12. Ulnar carpal bone
13. Accessory carpal bone
14. Carpal bone IV
15. Metacarpal bone V
16. Proximal sesamoid bone
17. Proximal phalanx of digit V
18. Middle phalanx of digit V
19. Distal phalanx of digit V
20. Distal sesamoid bone
21. Distal radial epiphysis
22. Intermedial carpal bone
23. Radial carpal bone
24. Carpal bones I to III
25. Metacarpal bones
26. Phalanges

B

Figure 7-13, A
Type of animal: Rabbit
Type of study: Thoracic limb
Projection: Ventrodorsal
Weight of animal: 2.2 kg
Gender: Male
Reproductive status: Neutered
Age: Adult

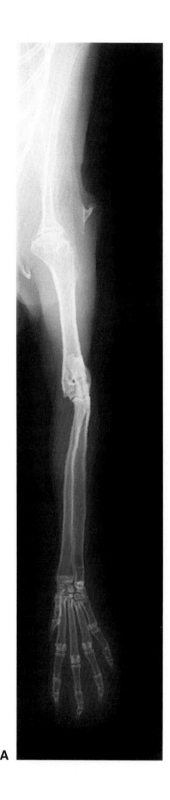

A

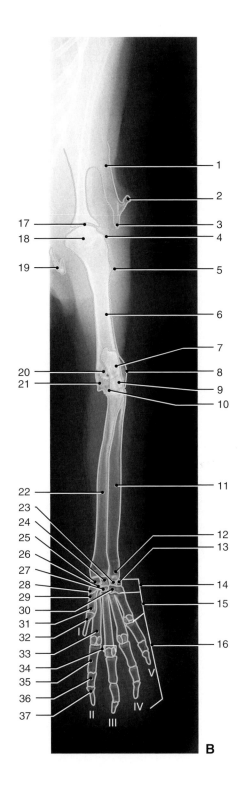

Figure 7-13, B
Type of animal: Rabbit
Type of study: Thoracic limb
Projection: Ventrodorsal
Weight of animal: 2.2 kg
Gender: Male
Reproductive status: Neutered
Age: Adult

1. Acromion
2. Suprahamate process
3. Hamate process
4. Greater tubercle of humerus
5. Deltoid tuberosity of humerus
6. Humerus
7. Olecranon of ulna
8. Lateral humeral epicondyle
9. Lateral humeral condyle
10. Humeroradial joint space
11. Ulna
12. Styloid process of ulna
13. Accessory carpal bone
14. Carpal bones
15. Metacarpal bones
16. Phalanges
17. Scapulohumeral joint space
18. Humeral head
19. Clavicle
20. Supratrochlear foramen of humerus
21. Medial humeral condyle
22. Radius
23. Ulnar carpal bone
24. Intermedial carpal bone
25. Radial carpal bone
26. Carpal bone II
27. Carpal bone III
28. Carpal bone I
29. Metacarpal bone I
30. Carpal bone IV
31. Proximal phalanx of digit I
32. Distal phalanx of digit I
33. Metacarpal bone II
34. Proximal sesamoid bones
35. Proximal phalanx of digit II
36. Middle phalanx of digit II
37. Distal phalanx of digit II

Figure 7-14, A
Type of animal: Rabbit
Type of study: Elbow joint
Projection: Mediolateral
Weight of animal: 3.4 kg
Gender: Female
Reproductive status: Intact
Age: Adult

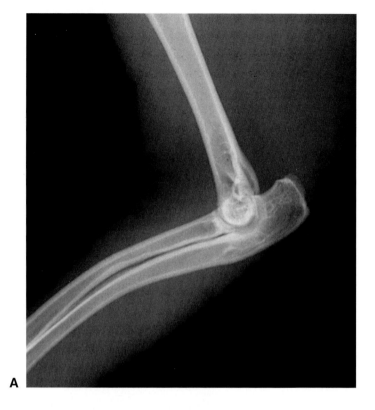

A

Figure 7-14, B
Type of animal: Rabbit
Type of study: Elbow joint
Projection: Mediolateral
Weight of animal: 3.4 kg
Gender: Female
Reproductive status: Intact
Age: Adult

1. Medial humeral epicondyle
2. Olecranon of ulna
3. Anconeal process of ulna
4. Trochlear notch of ulna
5. Ulna
6. Humerus
7. Humeral condyle
8. Humeroradial joint space
9. Radius

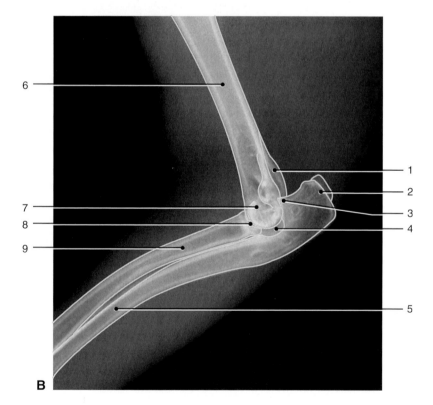

B

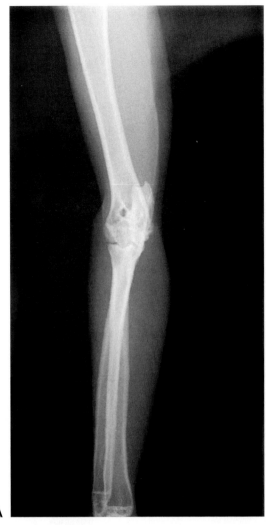

Figure 7-15, A
Type of animal: Rabbit
Type of study: Elbow joint
Projection: Caudocranial
Weight of animal: 3.4 kg
Gender: Female
Reproductive status: Intact
Age: Adult

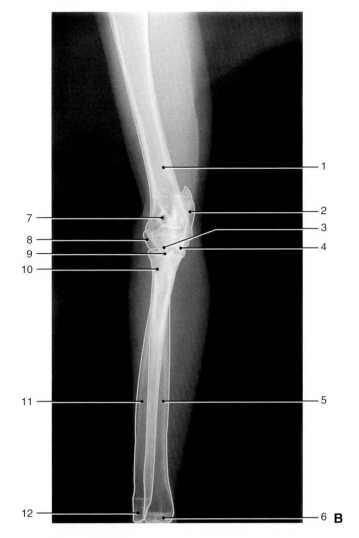

Figure 7-15, B
Type of animal: Rabbit
Type of study: Elbow joint
Projection: Caudocranial
Weight of animal: 3.4 kg
Gender: Female
Reproductive status: Intact
Age: Adult

1. Humerus
2. Olecranon of ulna
3. Lateral humeral condyle
4. Medial humeral condyle
5. Radius
6. Distal radial epiphysis
7. Supratrochlear foramen of humerus
8. Lateral humeral epicondyle
9. Humeroradial joint space
10. Proximal radius
11. Ulna
12. Styloid process of ulna

Figure 7-16, A
Type of animal: Rabbit
Type of study: Distal thoracic limb
Projection: Mediolateral
Weight of animal: 2.2 kg
Gender: Male
Reproductive status: Neutered
Age: Adult

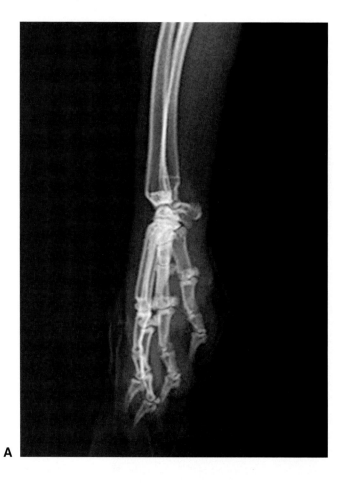

A

Figure 7-16, B
Type of animal: Rabbit
Type of study: Distal thoracic limb
Projection: Mediolateral
Weight of animal: 2.2 kg
Gender: Male
Reproductive status: Neutered
Age: Adult

1. Ulna
2. Styloid process of ulna
3. Ulnar carpal bone
4. Accessory carpal bone
5. Carpal bone IV
6. Metacarpal bone V
7. Proximal sesamoid bone
8. Proximal phalanx of digit V
9. Middle phalanx of digit V
10. Distal phalanx of digit V
11. Distal sesamoid bone
12. Radius
13. Distal radial epiphysis
14. Intermedial carpal bone
15. Radial carpal bone
16. Carpal bones I, II, and III
17. Metacarpal bones
18. Phalanges

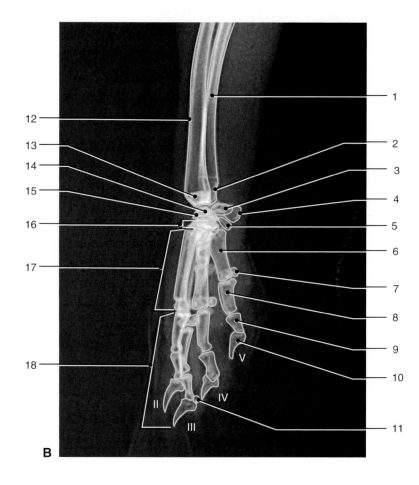

B

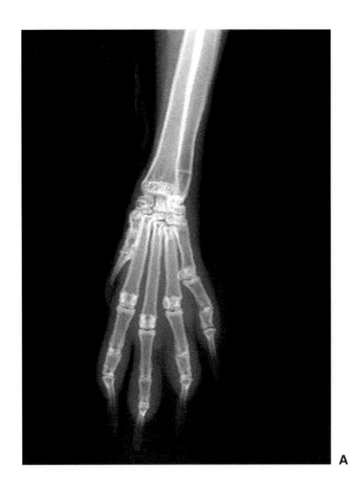

Figure 7-17, A
Type of animal: Rabbit
Type of study: Distal thoracic limb
Projection: Dorsopalmar
Weight of animal: 2.2 kg
Gender: Male
Reproductive status: Neutered
Age: Adult

A

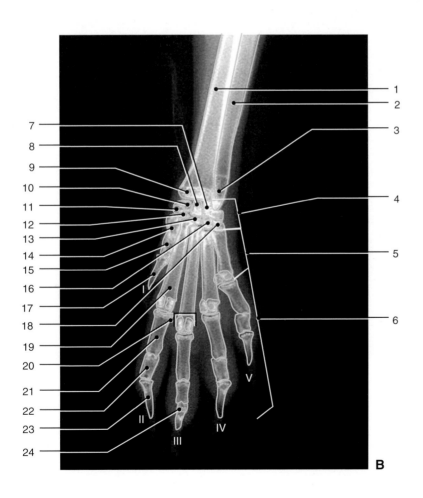

B

Figure 7-17, B
Type of animal: Rabbit
Type of study: Distal thoracic limb
Projection: Dorsopalmar
Weight of animal: 2.2 kg
Gender: Male
Reproductive status: Neutered
Age: Adult

1. Radius
2. Ulna
3. Styloid process of ulna
4. Carpal bones
5. Metacarpal bones
6. Phalanges
7. Accessory carpal bone
8. Ulnar carpal bone
9. Distal radial epiphysis
10. Intermedial carpal bone
11. Radial carpal bone
12. Carpal bone I
13. Carpal bone II
14. Metacarpal bone I
15. Proximal phalanx of digit I
16. Carpal bone III
17. Distal phalanx of digit I
18. Carpal bone IV
19. Metacarpal bone II
20. Proximal sesamoid bones
21. Proximal phalanx of digit II
22. Middle phalanx of digit II
23. Distal phalanx of digit II
24. Distal sesamoid bone

Figure 7-18, A
Type of animal: Rabbit
Type of study: Pelvis
Projection: Laterolateral
    (right lateral recumbency)
Weight of animal: 2.2 kg
Gender: Male
Reproductive status: Neutered
Age: Adult

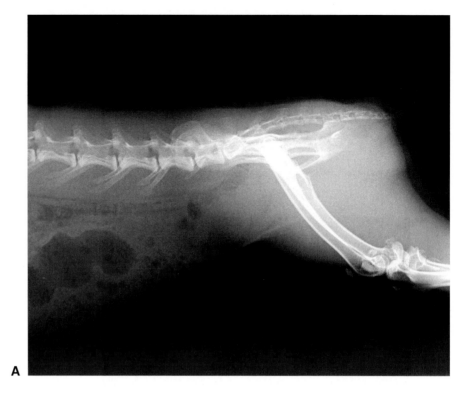

A

Figure 7-18, B
Type of animal: Rabbit
Type of study: Pelvis
Projection: Laterolateral
    (right lateral recumbency)
Weight of animal: 2.2 kg
Gender: Male
Reproductive status: Neutered
Age: Adult

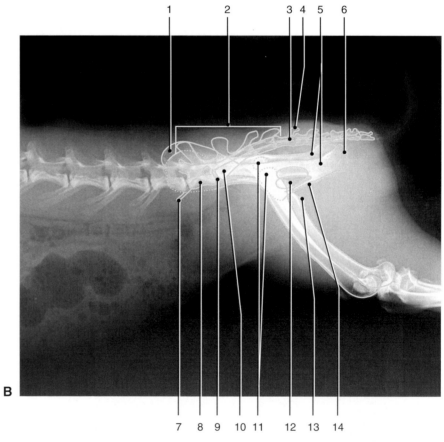

B

1. Ilium
2. Spinous processes of sacral vertebrae
3. 1st caudal vertebra
4. Articular process of caudal vertebra
5. Ischia
6. Ischial tuberosity
7. Transverse process of lumbar vertebra
8. 7th lumbar vertebra
9. Lumbosacral intervertebral space
10. Sacrum
11. Femoral heads
12. Obturator foramen
13. Lesser trochanter of femur
14. Pubis

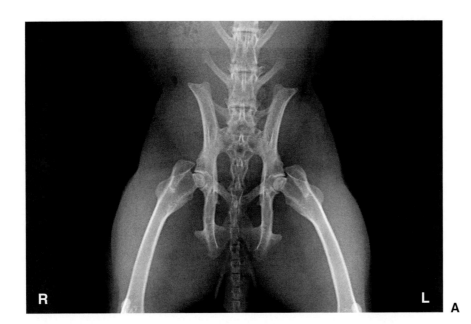

Figure 7-19, A
Type of animal: Rabbit
Type of study: Pelvis
Projection: Ventrodorsal
Weight of animal: 2.2 kg
Gender: Male
Reproductive status: Neutered
Age: Adult

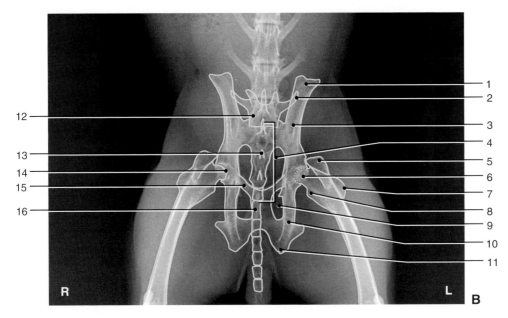

Figure 7-19, B
Type of animal: Rabbit
Type of study: Pelvis
Projection: Ventrodorsal
Weight of animal: 2.2 kg
Gender: Male
Reproductive status: Neutered
Age: Adult

1. Iliac crest
2. Transverse process of lumbar vertebra
3. Ilium
4. Sacrum
5. Greater trochanter of femur
6. Femoral head
7. 3rd trochanter of femur
8. Lesser trochanter of femur
9. Obturator foramen
10. Ischium
11. Ischial tuberosity
12. 7th lumbar vertebra
13. Spinous process of sacral vertebra
14. Acetabulum
15. Pubis
16. 1st caudal vertebra

Figure 7-20, A
Type of animal: Rabbit
Type of study: Pelvic limb
Projection: Mediolateral
Weight of animal: 2.2 kg
Gender: Male
Reproductive status: Neutered
Age: Adult

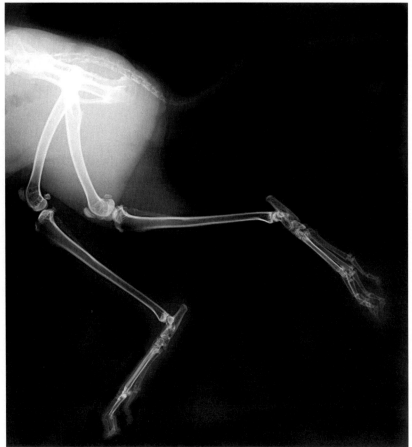

A

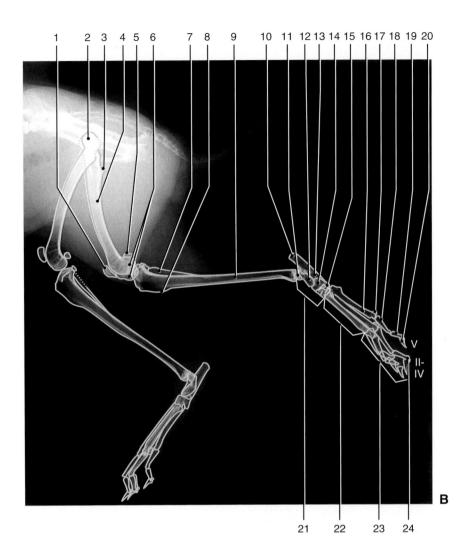

B

Figure 7-20, B
Type of animal: Rabbit
Type of study: Pelvic limb
Projection: Mediolateral
Weight of animal: 2.2 kg
Gender: Male
Reproductive status: Neutered
Age: Adult

1. Patella
2. Femoral head
3. Lesser trochanter of femur
4. Femur
5. Fabella
6. Femoral condyles
7. Fibula
8. Tibial crest
9. Tibia
10. Calcaneal tuber
11. Trochlea of talus
12. Talus
13. Calcaneus
14. Central tarsal bone
15. Tarsal bones II, III, and IV
16. Metatarsal bone V
17. Proximal sesamoid bone
18. Proximal phalanx of digit V
19. Middle phalanx of digit V
20. Distal phalanx of digit V
21. Tarsal bones
22. Metatarsal bones
23. Phalanges
24. Distal sesamoid bone

Figure 7-21, A
Type of animal: Rabbit
Type of study: Pelvic limb
Projection: Ventrodorsal
Weight of animal: 2.2 kg
Gender: Male
Reproductive status: Neutered
Age: Adult

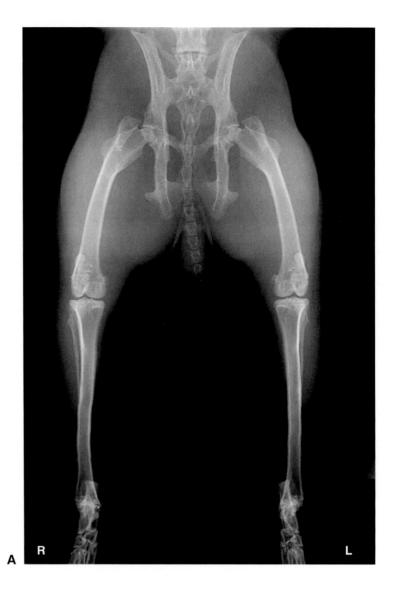

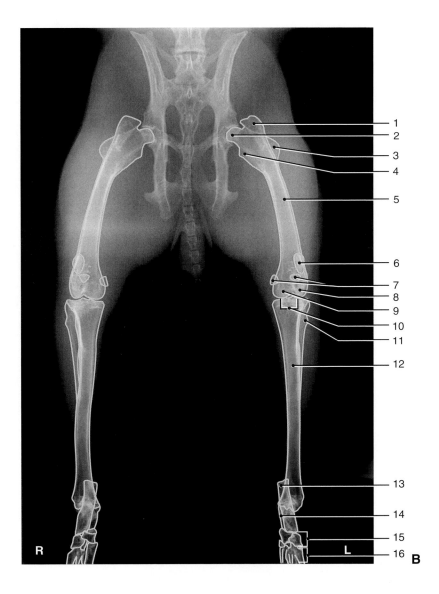

Figure 7-21, B
Type of animal: Rabbit
Type of study: Pelvic limb
Projection: Ventrodorsal
Weight of animal: 2.2 kg
Gender: Male
Reproductive status: Neutered
Age: Adult

1. Greater trochanter of femur
2. Femoral head
3. 3rd trochanter of femur
4. Lesser trochanter of femur
5. Femur
6. Patella
7. Fabellae
8. Lateral femoral condyle of femur
9. Medial femoral condyle of femur
10. Tibial intercondylar eminence
11. Fibula
12. Tibia
13. Calcaneal tuber
14. Talus
15. Tarsal bones
16. Metatarsal bones

Figure 7-22, A
Type of animal: Rabbit
Type of study: Stifle joint
Projection: Mediolateral
Weight of Animal: 2.2 kg
Gender: Male
Reproductive status: Neutered
Age: Adult

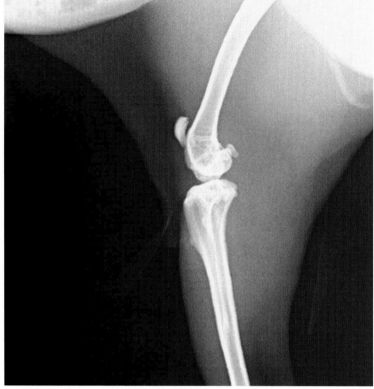

A

Figure 7-22, B
Type of animal: Rabbit
Type of study: Stifle joint
Projection: Mediolateral
Weight of animal: 2.2 kg
Gender: Male
Reproductive status: Neutered
Age: Adult

1. Femur
2. Fabellae
3. Medial femoral condyle
4. Fibula
5. Tibia
6. Patella
7. Femoral epicondyle
8. Lateral femoral condyle
9. Tibial crest

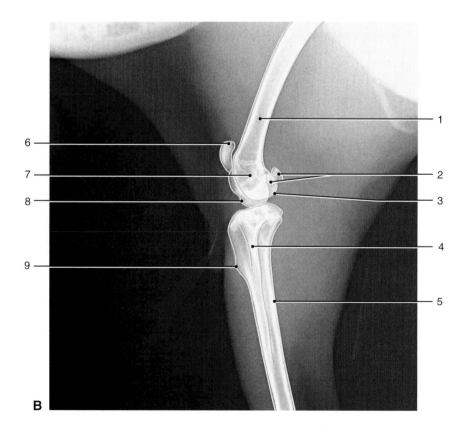

B

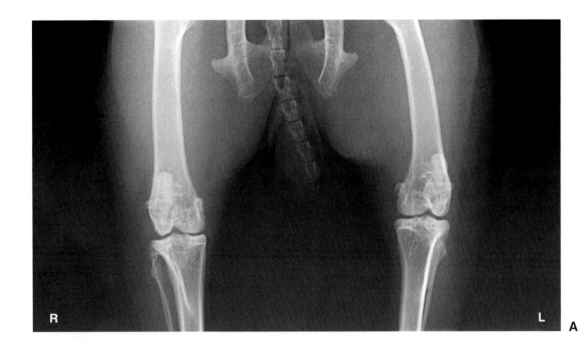

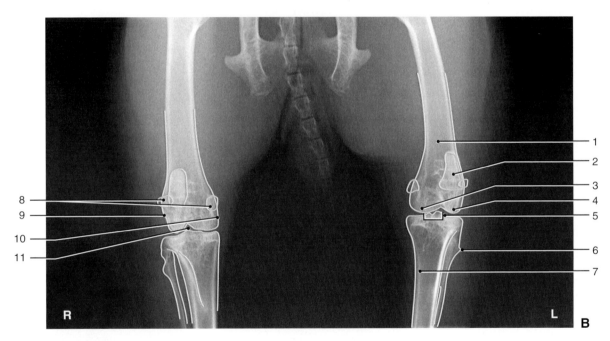

Figure 7-23

Type of animal: Rabbit
Type of study: Stifle joints
Projection: Craniocaudal
Weight of animal: 2.2 kg
Gender: Male
Reproductive status: Neutered
Age: Adult

1. Femur
2. Patella
3. Medial femoral condyle
4. Lateral femoral condyle
5. Tibial intercondylar eminence
6. Fibula

7. Tibia
8. Fabellae
9. Lateral femoral epicondyle
10. Medial femoral epicondyle
11. Femorotibial joint space

Figure 7-24, A
Type of animal: Rabbit
Type of study: Distal pelvic limb
Projection: Mediolateral
Weight of animal: 2.2 kg
Gender: Male
Reproductive status: Neutered
Age: Adult

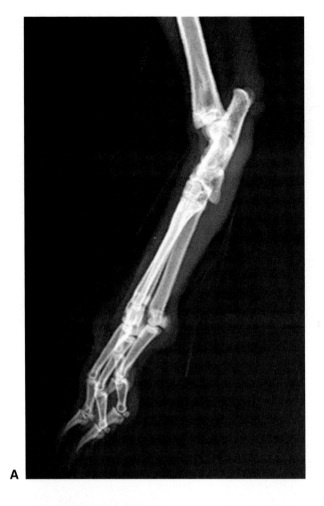

A

Figure 7-24, B
Type of animal: Rabbit
Type of study: Distal pelvic limb
Projection: Mediolateral
Weight of animal: 2.2 kg
Gender: Male
Reproductive status: Neutered
Age: Adult

1. Tibia
2. Calcaneal tuber
3. Lateral malleolus of fibula
4. Calcaneus
5. Trochlea of talus
6. Talus
7. Central tarsal bone
8. 3rd tarsal bone
9. Metatarsal bone
10. Proximal sesamoid bone
11. Proximal phalanx of digit II
12. Middle phalanx of digit II
13. Distal sesamoid bone
14. Distal phalanx of digit II
15. Tarsal bones
16. Metatarsal bones
17. Phalanges

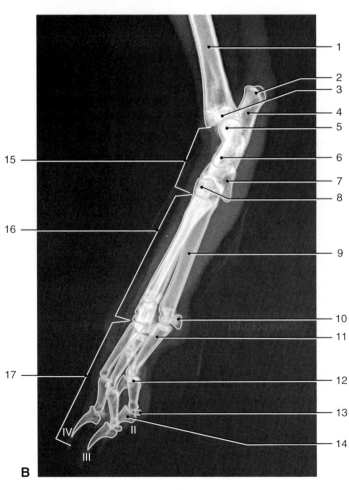

B

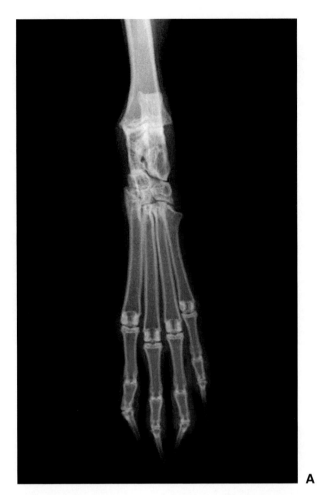

A

Figure 7-25, A
Type of animal: Rabbit
Type of study: Distal pelvic limb
Projection: Dorsoplantar
Weight of animal: 2.2 kg
Gender: Male
Reproductive status: Neutered
Age: Adult

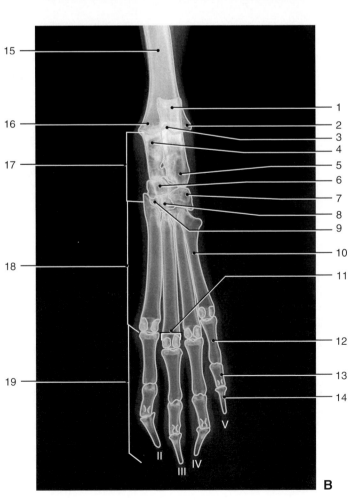

B

Figure 7-25, B
Type of animal: Rabbit
Type of study: Distal pelvic limb
Projection: Dorsoplantar
Weight of animal: 2.2 kg
Gender: Male
Reproductive status: Neutered
Age: Adult

1. Calcaneal tuber
2. Lateral malleolus of fibula
3. Tibiotarsal joint space
4. Talus
5. Calcaneus
6. Central tarsal bone
7. Tarsal bone IV
8. Tarsal bone III
9. Tarsal bone II
10. Metatarsal bone V
11. Proximal sesamoid bones
12. Proximal phalanx of digit V
13. Middle phalanx of digit V
14. Distal phalanx of digit V
15. Tibia
16. Medial malleolus of tibia
17. Tarsal bones
18. Metatarsal bones
19. Phalanges

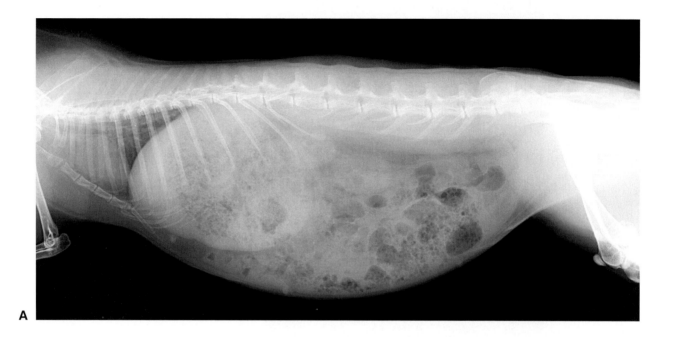

A

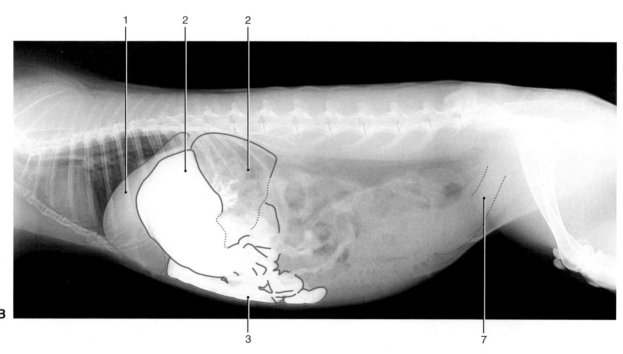

B

Figure 7-26, A-E
Type of animal: Rabbit
Type of study: Gastrointestinal positive contrast study
Contrast medium: Barium sulfate suspension
  (Novopaque 60% w/v; Lafayette Pharmaceutical,
  Inc., Lafayette, Ind.) 60 ml administered per os
Projection: Laterolateral (right lateral recumbency)
Weight of animal: 4.1 kg
Gender: Female
Reproductive status: Intact
Age: Adult

1. Liver
2. Stomach
3. Small intestine
4. Cecum
5. Ileum
6. Vermiform appendix
7. Urinary bladder
8. Right kidney
9. Left kidney
10. Colon

Image	Time (hr)
A	Survey
B	0.5

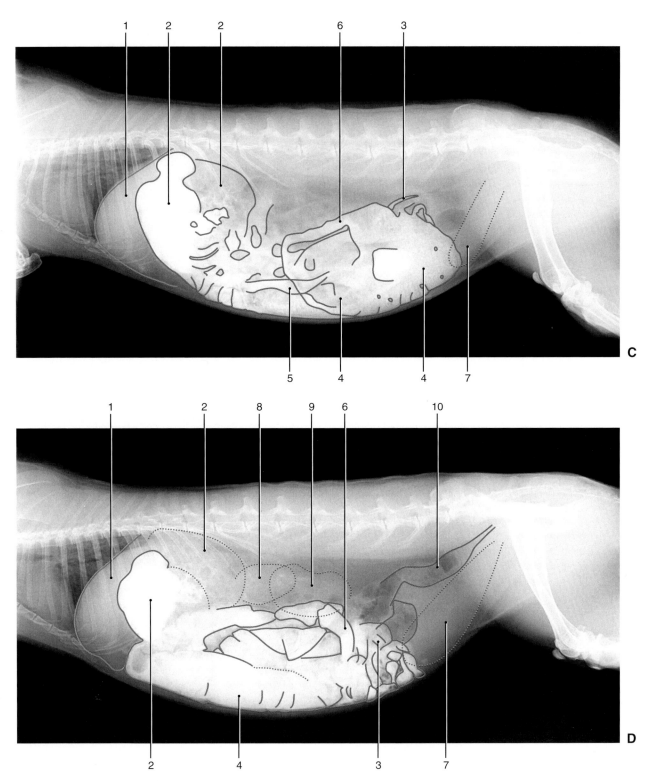

Figure 7-26, A-E—cont'd
Type of animal: Rabbit
Type of study: Gastrointestinal positive contrast study
Contrast medium: Barium sulfate suspension
   (Novopaque 60% w/v; Lafayette Pharmaceutical,
   Inc., Lafayette, Ind.) 60 ml administered per os
Projection: Laterolateral (right lateral recumbency)
Weight of animal: 4.1 kg
Gender: Female
Reproductive status: Intact
Age: Adult

1. Liver
2. Stomach
3. Small intestine
4. Cecum
5. Ileum
6. Vermiform appendix
7. Urinary bladder
8. Right kidney
9. Left kidney
10. Colon

Image	Time (hr)
C	1.5
D	3.0

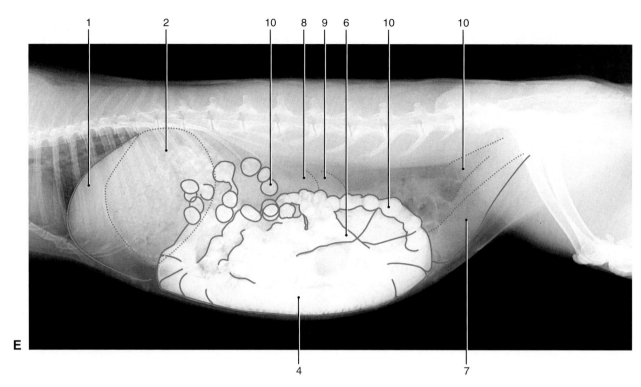

Figure 7-26, A-E—cont'd
Type of animal: Rabbit
Type of study: Gastrointestinal positive contrast study
Contrast medium: Barium sulfate suspension
(Novopaque 60% w/v; Lafayette Pharmaceutical,
Inc., Lafayette, Ind.) 60 ml administered per os
Projection: Laterolateral (right lateral recumbency)
Weight of animal: 4.1 kg
Gender: Female
Reproductive status: Intact
Age: Adult

1. Liver
2. Stomach
3. Small intestine
4. Cecum
5. Ileum
6. Vermiform appendix
7. Urinary bladder
8. Right kidney
9. Left kidney
10. Colon

Image	Time (hr)
E	6.0

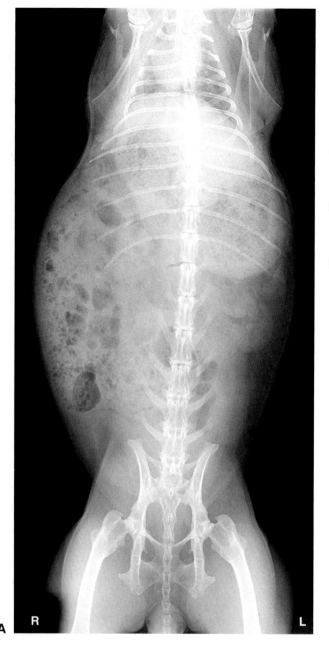

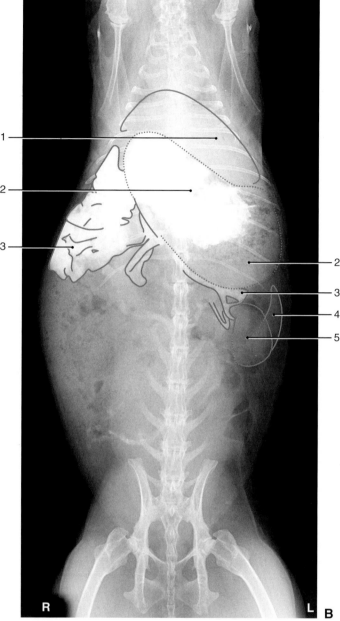

Figure 7-27, A-E
Type of animal: Rabbit
Type of study: Gastrointestinal positive contrast study
Contrast medium: Barium sulfate suspension (Novopaque
    60% w/v; Lafayette Pharmaceutical, Inc., Lafayette, Ind.)
    60 ml administered per os
Projection: Ventrodorsal
Weight of animal: 4.1 kg
Gender: Female
Reproductive status: Intact
Age: Adult

1. Liver
2. Stomach
3. Small intestine
4. Spleen
5. Left kidney
6. Vermiform appendix
7. Cecum
8. Ileum
9. Colon

Image	Time (hr)
A	Survey
B	0.5

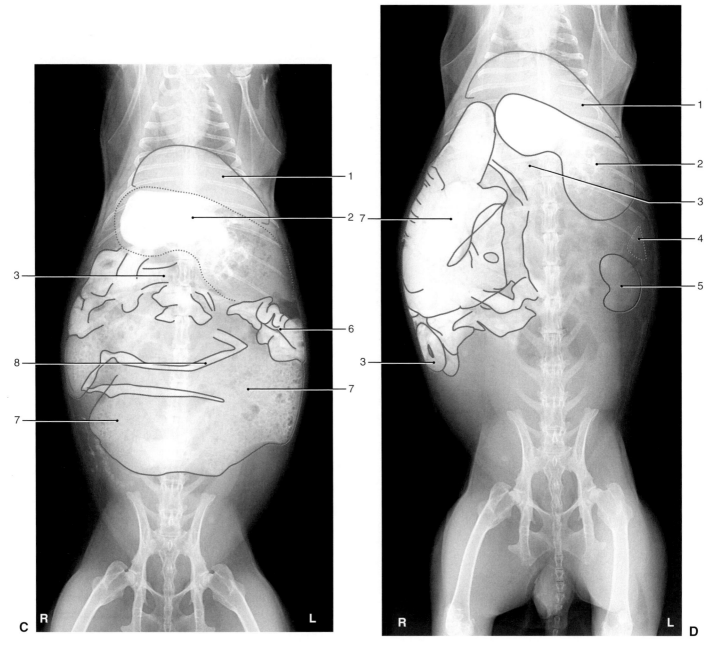

Figure 7-27, A-E—cont'd
Type of animal: Rabbit
Type of study: Gastrointestinal positive contrast study
Contrast medium: Barium sulfate suspension (Novopaque
   60% w/v; Lafayette Pharmaceutical, Inc., Lafayette, Ind.)
   60 ml administered per os
Projection: Ventrodorsal
Weight of animal: 4.1 kg
Gender: Female
Reproductive status: Intact
Age: Adult

1. Liver
2. Stomach
3. Small intestine
4. Spleen
5. Left kidney
6. Vermiform appendix
7. Cecum
8. Ileum
9. Colon

Image	Time (hr)
C	1.5
D	3.0

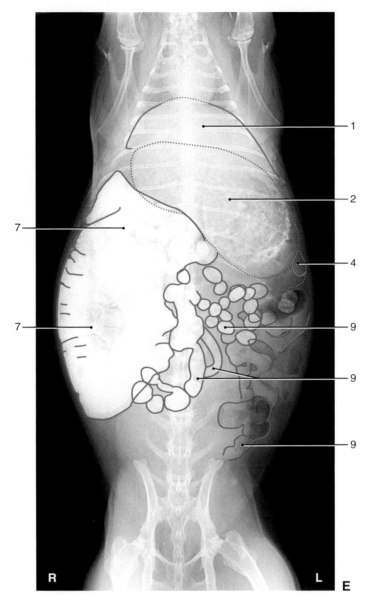

Figure 7-27, A-E—cont'd
Type of animal: Rabbit
Type of study: Gastrointestinal positive contrast study
Contrast medium: Barium sulfate suspension (Novopaque
    60% w/v; Lafayette Pharmaceutical, Inc., Lafayette, Ind.)
    60 ml administered per os
Projection: Ventrodorsal
Weight of animal: 4.1 kg
Gender: Female
Reproductive status: Intact
Age: Adult

Image	Time (hr)
E	6.0

1. Liver
2. Stomach
3. Small intestine
4. Spleen
5. Left kidney
6. Vermiform appendix
7. Cecum
8. Ileum
9. Colon

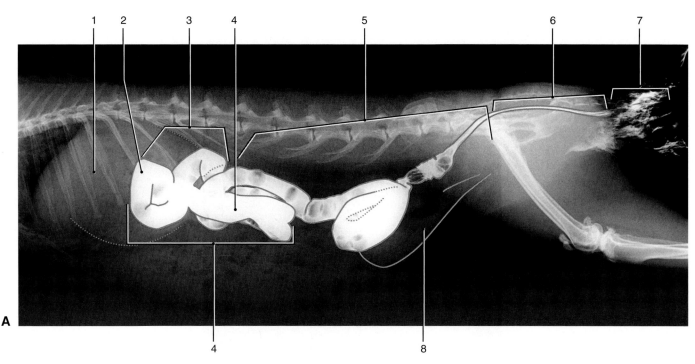

Figure 7-28, A

Type of animal: Rabbit
Type of study: Double contrast barium enema
Contrast medium: Barium sulfate suspension (Novopaque
    60% w/v; Lafayette Pharmaceutical, Inc., Lafayette, Ind.)
    80 ml administered per rectum
Projection: Laterolateral (right lateral recumbency)
Weight of animal: 3.5 kg
Gender: Female
Reproductive status: Intact
Age: Adult

1. Stomach
2. Hepatic flexure of colon
3. Transverse colon
4. Ascending colon
5. Descending colon
6. Rectum
7. Positive contrast medium on hair
8. Urinary bladder

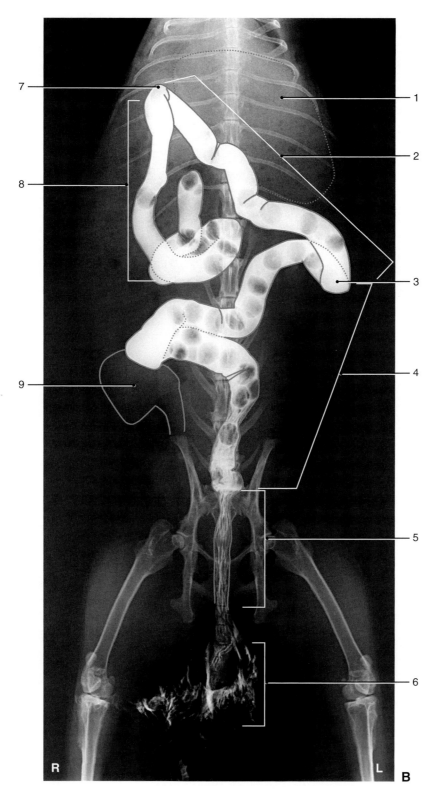

Figure 7-28, B

Type of animal: Rabbit
Type of study: Double contrast barium enema
Contrast medium: Barium sulfate suspension
    (Novopaque 60% w/v; Lafayette Pharmaceutical,
    Inc., Lafayette, Ind.) 80 ml administered per rectum
Projection: Ventrodorsal
Weight of animal: 3.5 kg
Gender: Female
Reproductive status: Intact
Age: Adult

1. Stomach
2. Transverse colon
3. Splenic flexure of colon
4. Descending colon
5. Rectum
6. Positive contrast
    medium on hair
7. Hepatic flexure of colon
8. Ascending colon
9. Urinary bladder

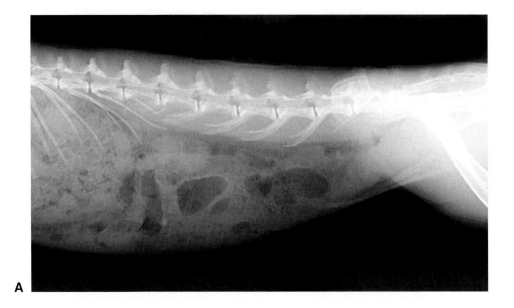

A

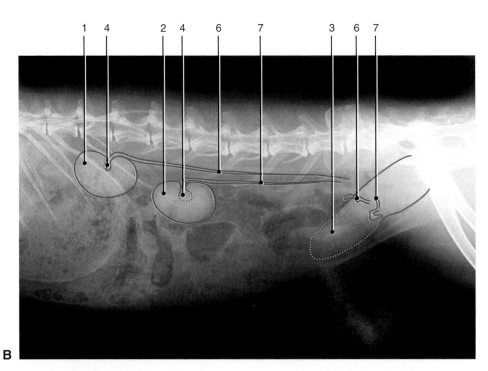

B

Figure 7-29, A-D
Type of animal: Rabbit
Type of study: Excretory urogram
Contrast medium: RenoCal-76 (37% organically bound iodine; Bracco Diagnostics, Inc., Princeton, NJ) 9 ml IV (3 ml/kg)
Projection: Laterolateral (right lateral recumbency)
Weight of animal: 3.2 kg
Gender: Female
Reproductive status: Intact
Age: Adult

1. Right kidney
2. Left kidney
3. Urinary bladder
4. Renal pelvis
5. Recesses of renal pelvis
6. Right ureter
7. Left ureter
8. Compression bandage

Image	Time (min)
A	Survey
B	1.0*

*Compression bandage applied 20 min after image B was obtained.

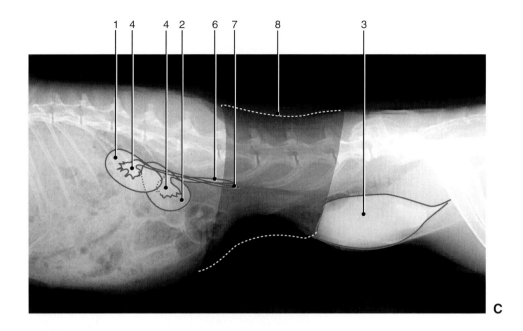

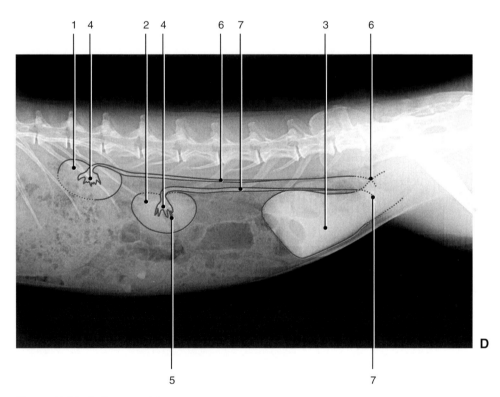

Figure 7-29, A-D—cont'd

Type of animal: Rabbit
Type of study: Excretory urogram
Contrast medium: RenoCal-76 (37% organically bound
    iodine; Bracco Diagnostics, Inc., Princeton, NJ) 9 ml IV
    (3 ml/kg)
Projection: Laterolateral (right lateral recumbency)
Weight of animal: 3.2 kg
Gender: Female
Reproductive status: Intact
Age: Adult

1. Right kidney
2. Left kidney
3. Urinary bladder
4. Renal pelvis
5. Recesses of renal pelvis
6. Right ureter
7. Left ureter
8. Compression bandage

Image	Time (min)
C	40.0*
D	45.0

*Compression bandage removed after image C was obtained.

Figure 7-30, A-E
Type of animal: Rabbit
Type of study: Excretory urogram
Projection: Ventrodorsal
Contrast medium: RenoCal-76 (37% organically
  bound iodine; Bracco Diagnostics, Inc.,
  Princeton, NJ) 9 ml IV (3 ml/kg)
Weight of animal: 3.2 kg
Gender: Female
Reproductive status: Intact
Age: Adult

Image	Time (min)
A	Survey
B	1.0*

*Compression bandage applied 20 min after
image B was obtained.

1. Right kidney
2. Left kidney
3. Urinary bladder
4. Renal pelvis
5. Recesses of renal pelvis
6. Right ureter
7. Left ureter
8. Compression bandage

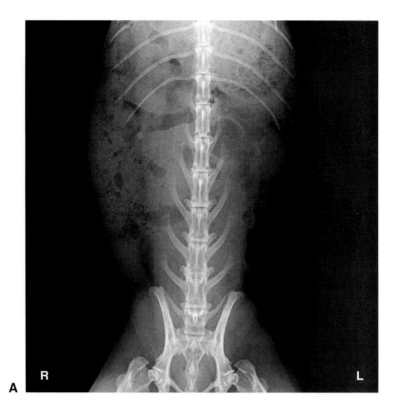

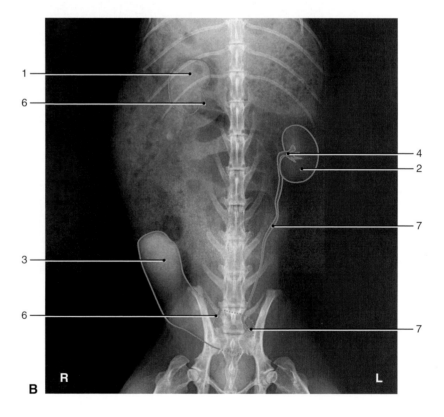

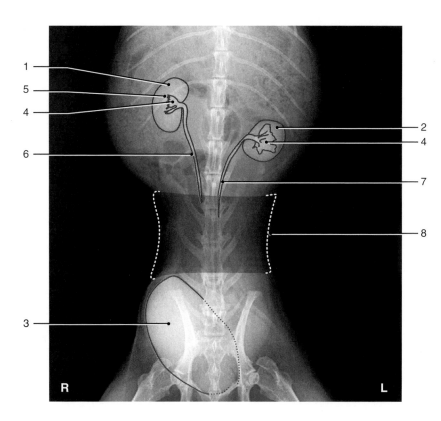

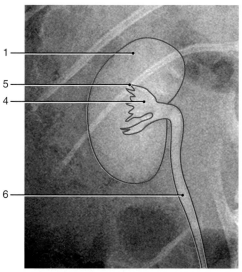

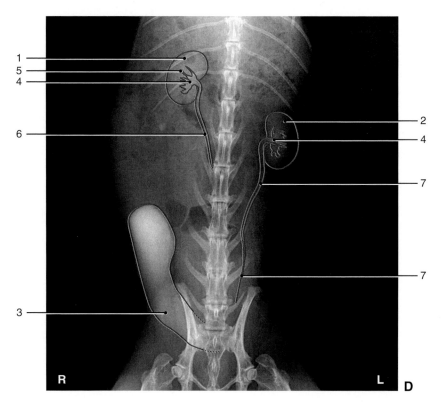

Figure 7-30, A-E—cont'd
Type of animal: Rabbit
Type of study: Excretory urogram
Projection: Ventrodorsal
Contrast medium: RenoCal-76 (37% organically
   bound iodine; Bracco Diagnostics, Inc.,
   Princeton, NJ) 9 ml IV (3 ml/kg)
Weight of animal: 3.2 kg
Gender: Female
Reproductive status: Intact
Age: Adult

Image	Time (min)
C	40.0*
D	45.0
E	40.0*

*Compression bandage removed after
images C and E were obtained.

1. Right kidney
2. Left kidney
3. Urinary bladder
4. Renal pelvis
5. Recesses of renal pelvis
6. Right ureter
7. Left ureter
8. Compression bandage

Figure 7-31, A-D
Type of animal: Rabbit
Type of study: Double contrast retrograde cystogram
Contrast medium: RenoCal-76 (37% organically
    bound iodine; Bracco Diagnostics, Inc., Princeton, NJ)
    2 ml administered via urinary catheter; 1 ml of fluid
    in bladder removed after administration of
    RenoCal-76; 35 ml of air administered via
    urinary catheter
Projection: Laterolateral (right lateral recumbency)
Weight of animal: 3.2 kg
Gender: Female
Reproductive status: Intact
Age: Adult

Image	Projection
A	Laterolateral survey
B	Laterolateral double contrast retrograde cystogram

1. Body of urinary bladder
2. Neck of urinary bladder
3. Urinary catheter
4. Wall of urinary bladder
5. Gas-filled lumen of urinary bladder
6. Positive contrast medium

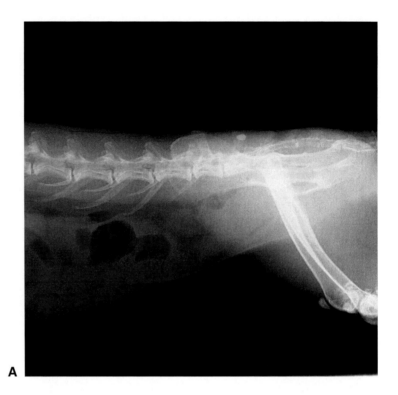

A

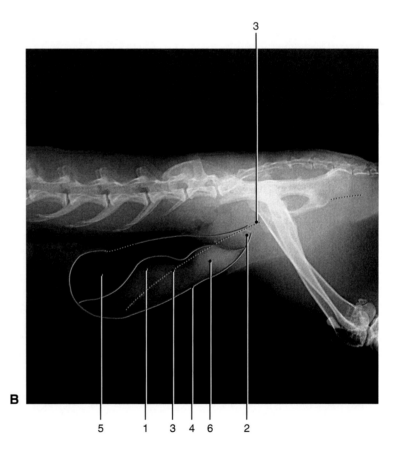

B

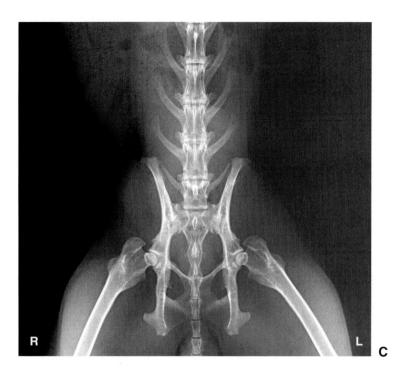

Figure 7-31, A-D—cont'd
Type of animal: Rabbit
Type of study: Double contrast retrograde cystogram
Contrast medium: RenoCal-76 (37% organically
   bound iodine; Bracco Diagnostics, Inc., Princeton, NJ)
   2 ml administered via urinary catheter; 1 ml of fluid
   in bladder removed after administration of
   RenoCal-76; 35 ml of air administered via
   urinary catheter
Projection: Ventrodorsal
Weight of animal: 3.2 kg
Gender: Female
Reproductive status: Intact
Age: Adult

Image	Projection
C	Ventrodorsal survey
D	Ventrodorsal oblique double contrast retrograde cystogram

1. Body of urinary bladder
2. Neck of urinary bladder
3. Urinary catheter
4. Wall of urinary bladder
5. Gas-filled lumen of urinary bladder
6. Positive contrast medium

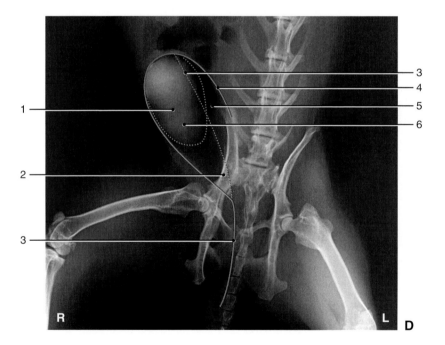

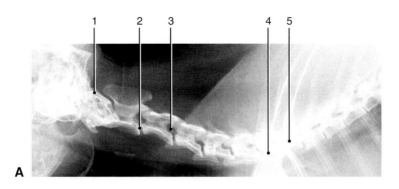

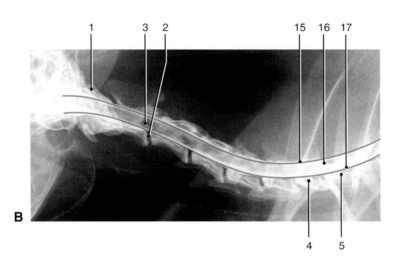

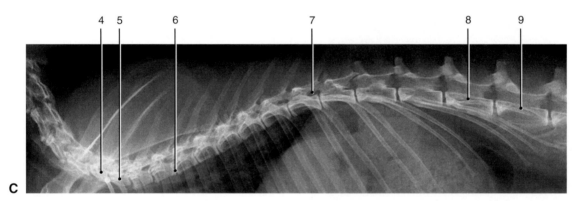

Figure 7-32, A-F
Type of animal: Rabbit
Type of study: Myelogram
Contrast medium: Isovue 200 (iopamidol injection 41%, 20% bound iodine; Bracco Diagnostics, Inc., Princeton, NJ); injection site L5-L6
Projection: Laterolateral (right lateral recumbency)
Weight of animal: 3.5 kg
Gender: Female
Reproductive status: Intact
Age: Adult

1. Atlas
2. Cervical intervertebral space
3. Cervical intervertebral foramen
4. 7th cervical vertebra
5. 1st thoracic vertebra
6. Thoracic intervertebral space
7. Thoracic intervertebral foramen
8. 13th thoracic vertebra
9. 1st lumbar vertebra
10. Lumbar intervertebral space
11. Articular processes of lumbar vertebrae
12. Lumbar intervertebral foramen
13. 7th lumbar vertebra
14. Sacrum
15. Dorsal aspect of subarachnoid space
16. Spinal cord
17. Ventral aspect of subarachnoid space
18. Spinal needle

Image	Projection
A	Cervical vertebral column survey
B	Cervical vertebral column myelogram
C	Thoracic vertebral column survey

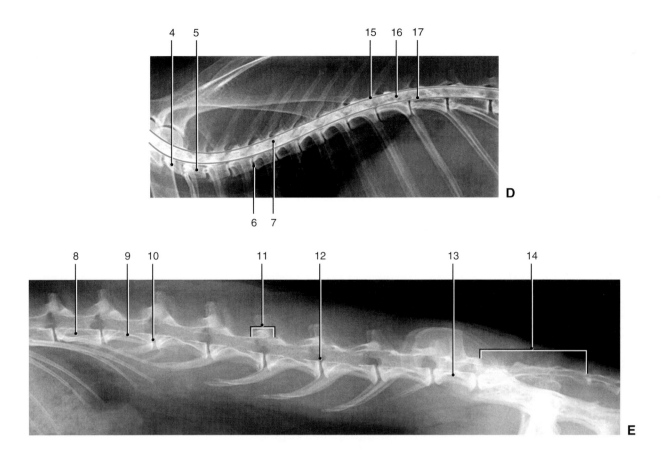

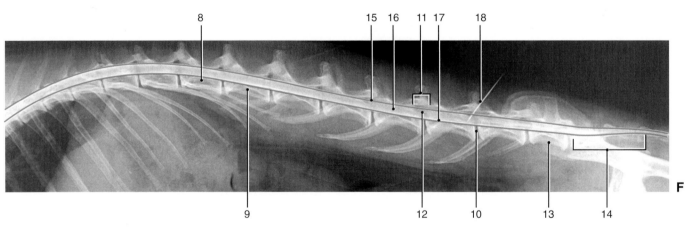

Figure 7-32, A-F—cont'd
Type of animal: Rabbit
Type of study: Myelogram
Contrast medium: Isovue 200 (iopamidol injection 41%,
    20% bound iodine; Bracco Diagnostics, Inc., Princeton,
    NJ); injection site L5-L6
Projection: Laterolateral (right lateral recumbency)
Weight of animal: 3.5 kg
Gender: Female
Reproductive status: Intact
Age: Adult

1. Atlas
2. Cervical intervertebral space
3. Cervical intervertebral foramen
4. 7th cervical vertebra
5. 1st thoracic vertebra
6. Thoracic intervertebral space
7. Thoracic intervertebral foramen
8. 13th thoracic vertebra
9. 1st lumbar vertebra
10. Lumbar intervertebral space
11. Articular processes of lumbar vertebrae
12. Lumbar intervertebral foramen
13. 7th lumbar vertebra
14. Sacrum
15. Dorsal aspect of subarachnoid space
16. Spinal cord
17. Ventral aspect of subarachnoid space
18. Spinal needle

Image	Projection
D	Thoracic vertebral column myelogram
E	Lumbar vertebral column survey
F	Lumbar vertebral column myelogram

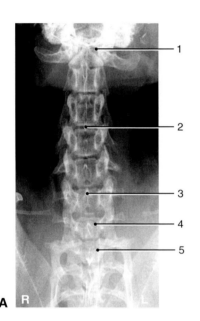

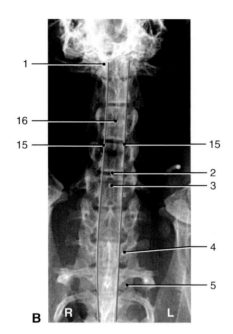

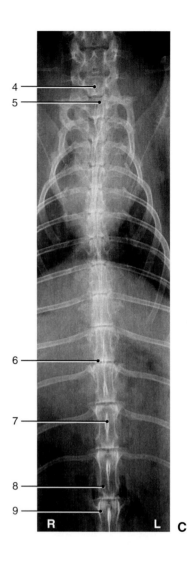

Figure 7-33, A-F
Type of animal: Rabbit
Type of study: Myelogram
Contrast medium: Isovue 200 (iopamidol injection 41%,
    20% bound iodine; Bracco Diagnostics, Inc., Princeton,
    NJ); injection site L5-L6
Projection: Dorsoventral
Weight of animal: 3.5 kg
Gender: Female
Reproductive status: Intact
Age: Adult

Image	Projection
A	Cervical vertebral column survey
B	Cervical vertebral column myelogram
C	Thoracic vertebral column survey

1. Atlas
2. Cervical intervertebral space
3. Spinous process of cervical vertebra
4. 7th cervical vertebra
5. 1st thoracic vertebra
6. Thoracic intervertebral space
7. Spinous process of thoracic vertebra
8. 13th thoracic vertebra
9. 1st lumbar vertebra
10. Lumbar intervertebral space
11. Spinous process of lumbar vertebra
12. Articular processes of lumbar vertebrae
13. 7th lumbar vertebra
14. Sacrum
15. Lateral aspect of subarachnoid space
16. Spinal cord

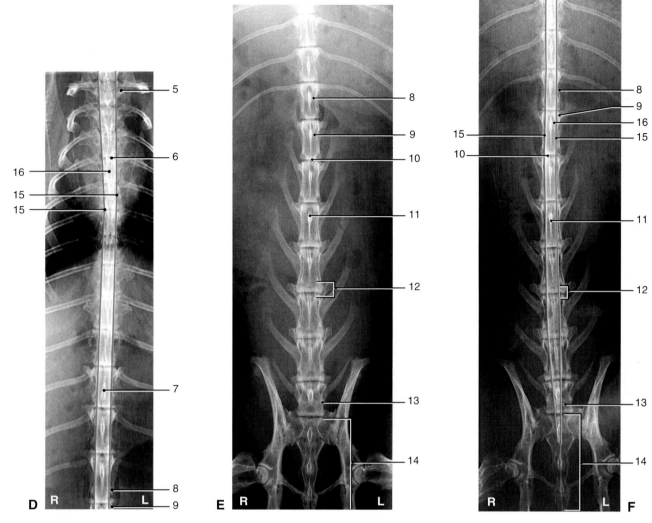

Figure 7-33, A-F—cont'd
Type of animal: Rabbit
Type of study: Myelogram
Contrast medium: Isovue 200 (iopamidol injection 41%,
   20% bound iodine; Bracco Diagnostics, Inc., Princeton,
   NJ); injection site L5-L6
Projection: Dorsoventral
Weight of animal: 3.5 kg
Gender: Female
Reproductive status: Intact
Age: Adult

Image	Projection
D	Thoracic vertebral column myelogram
E	Lumbar vertebral column survey
F	Lumbar vertebral column myelogram

1. Atlas
2. Cervical intervertebral space
3. Spinous process of cervical vertebra
4. 7th cervical vertebra
5. 1st thoracic vertebra
6. Thoracic intervertebral space
7. Spinous process of thoracic vertebra
8. 13th thoracic vertebra
9. 1st lumbar vertebra
10. Lumbar intervertebral space
11. Spinous process of lumbar vertebra
12. Articular processes of lumbar vertebrae
13. 7th lumbar vertebra
14. Sacrum
15. Lateral aspect of subarachnoid space
16. Spinal cord

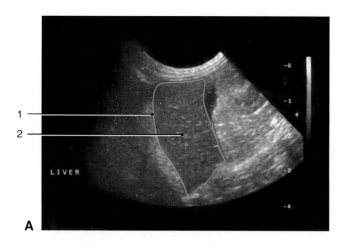

Figure 7-34, A
Sagittal image of liver

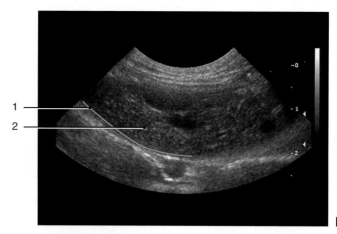

Figure 7-34, B
Transverse image of liver

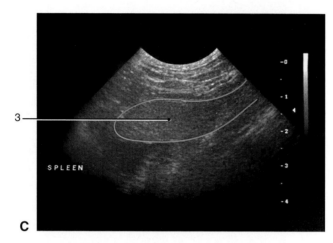

Figure 7-34, C
Sagittal image of spleen

Figure 7-34, A-C
Type of animal: Rabbit
Type of study: Ultrasound study of liver and spleen
Weight of animal: 3.2 kg
Gender: Female
Reproductive status: Intact
Age: Adult

1. Diaphragm
2. Liver
3. Spleen

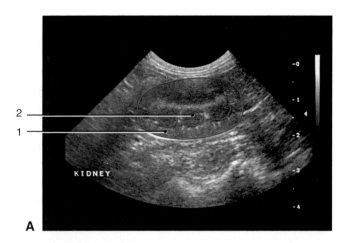

Figure 7-35, A
Sagittal image of left kidney

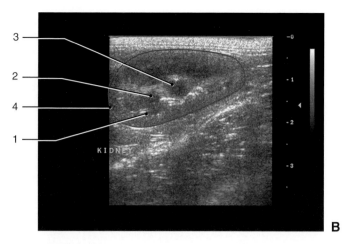

Figure 7-35, B
Sagittal image of left kidney

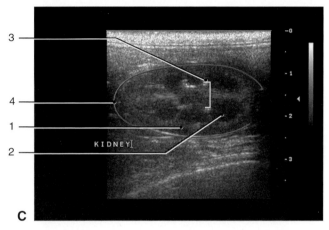

Figure 7-35, C
Sagittal image of left kidney

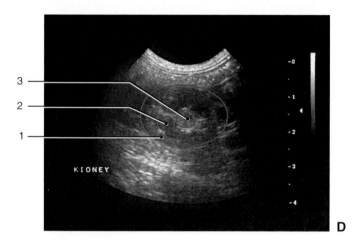

Figure 7-35, D
Transverse image of left kidney

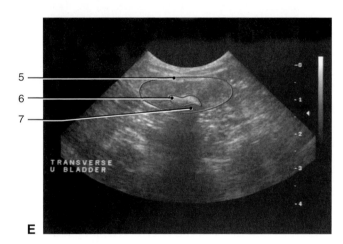

Figure 7-35, E
Transverse image of urinary bladder

Figure 7-35, A-E
Type of animal: Rabbit
Type of study: Ultrasound study of urinary tract
Weight of animal: 3.2 kg
Gender: Female
Reproductive status: Intact
Age: Adult

1. Renal cortex
2. Renal medulla
3. Renal pelvis
4. Cranial pole of kidney
5. Ventral aspect of urinary bladder wall
6. Lumen of urinary bladder (debris filled)
7. Dorsal aspect of urinary bladder wall

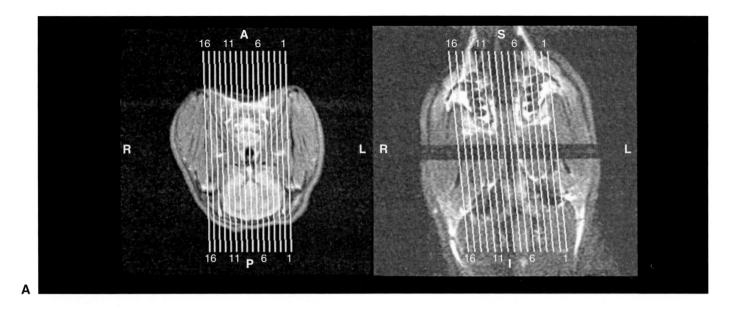

A

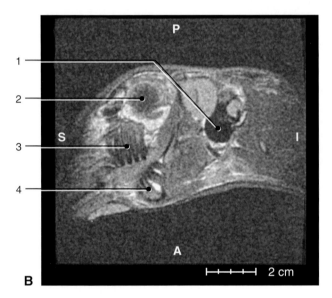

B

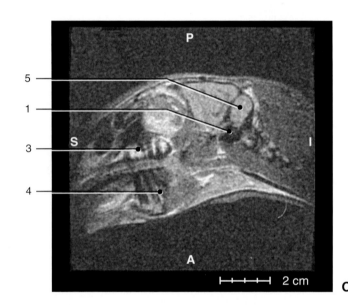

C

Figure 7-36, A-E

Type of animal: Rabbit
Type of study: MRI head
Imaging plane: Sagittal
Gender: Male
Reproductive status: Intact
Age: Adult

1. Tympanic cavity
2. Eyeball
3. Maxillary molar tooth
4. Mandibular molar tooth
5. Cerebellum
6. Cerebrum

7. Olfactory bulb
8. Basisphenoidal bone
9. Tongue
10. Brain stem
11. Spinal cord
12. Pharynx

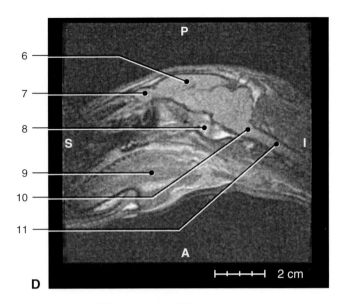

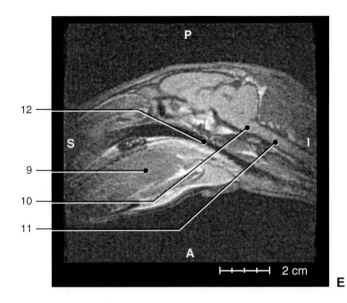

Figure 7-36, A-E—cont'd

Type of animal: Rabbit
Type of study: MRI head
Imaging plane: Sagittal
Gender: Male
Reproductive status: Intact
Age: Adult

1. Tympanic cavity
2. Eyeball
3. Maxillary molar tooth
4. Mandibular molar tooth
5. Cerebellum
6. Cerebrum

7. Olfactory bulb
8. Basisphenoidal bone
9. Tongue
10. Brain stem
11. Spinal cord
12. Pharynx

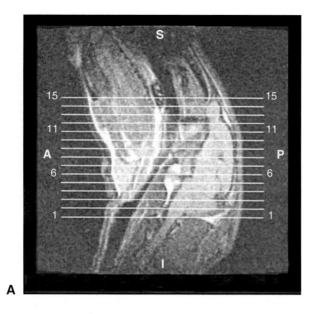

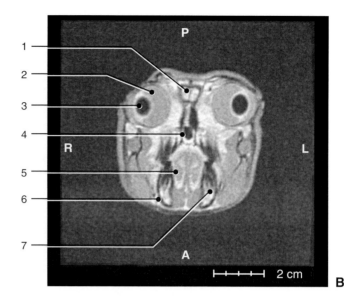

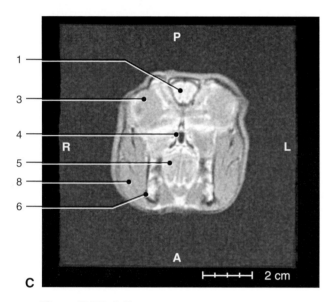

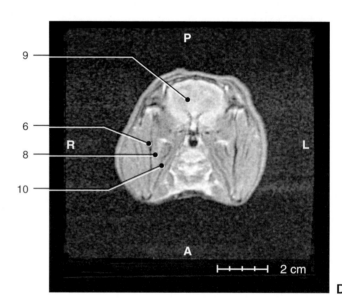

Figure 7-37, A-F

Type of animal: Rabbit
Type of study: MRI head
Imaging plane: Transverse
Gender: Male
Reproductive status: Intact
Age: Adult

1. Olfactory bulb
2. Eyeball
3. Lens of eyeball
4. Nasopharynx
5. Tongue
6. Mandible
7. Mandibular molar teeth
8. Masseter muscle
9. Cerebrum

10. Pterygoid muscle
11. Thalamus
12. Tympanic cavity
13. 3rd ventricle
14. Basisphenoidal bone
15. Cerebellum
16. Ear canal
17. Larynx

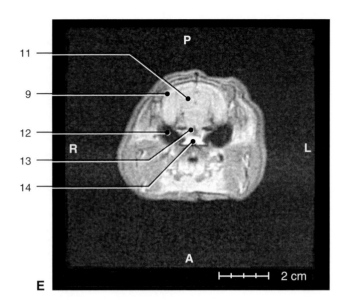

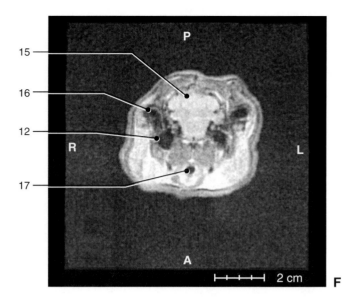

Figure 7-37, A-F—cont'd

Type of animal: Rabbit
Type of study: MRI head
Imaging plane: Transverse
Gender: Male
Reproductive status: Intact
Age: Adult

1. Olfactory bulb
2. Eyeball
3. Lens of eyeball
4. Nasopharynx
5. Tongue
6. Mandible
7. Mandibular molar teeth
8. Masseter muscle
9. Cerebrum

10. Pterygoid muscle
11. Thalamus
12. Tympanic cavity
13. 3rd ventricle
14. Basisphenoidal bone
15. Cerebellum
16. Ear canal
17. Larynx

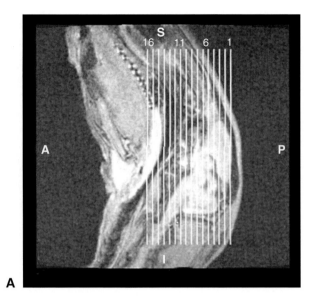

A

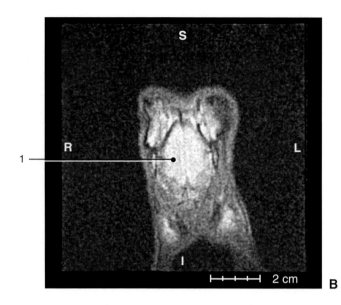

B

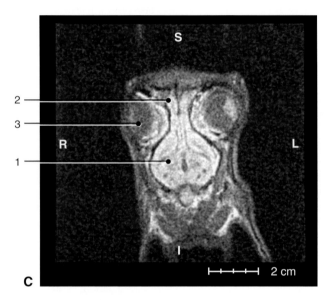

C

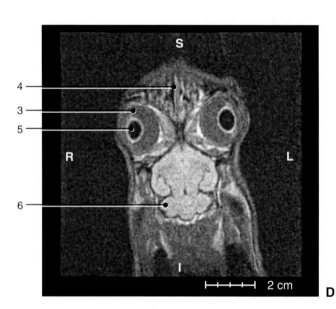

D

Figure 7-38, A-F

Type of animal: Rabbit
Type of study: MRI head
Imaging plane: Coronal
Gender: Male
Reproductive status: Intact
Age: Adult

1. Cerebrum
2. Olfactory bulb
3. Eyeball
4. Ethmoturbinates
5. Lens of eyeball
6. Cerebellum
7. Nasal cavity

8. Brain stem
9. Molar teeth
10. Mandible
11. Masseter muscle
12. Pterygoid muscle
13. Tympanic cavity

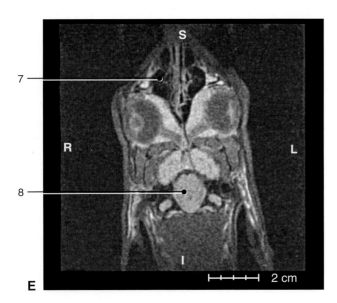

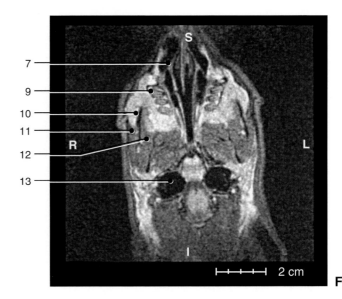

Figure 7-38, A-F—cont'd
Type of animal: Rabbit
Type of study: MRI head
Imaging plane: Coronal
Gender: Male
Reproductive status: Intact
Age: Adult

1. Cerebrum
2. Olfactory bulb
3. Eyeball
4. Ethmoturbinates
5. Lens of eyeball
6. Cerebellum
7. Nasal cavity

8. Brain stem
9. Molar teeth
10. Mandible
11. Masseter muscle
12. Pterygoid muscle
13. Tympanic cavity

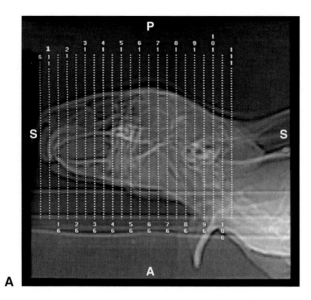

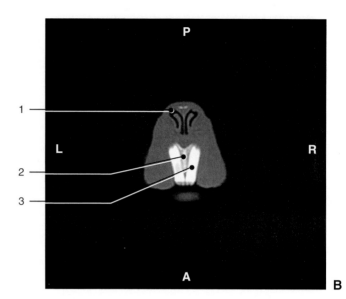

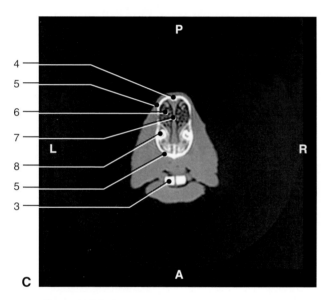

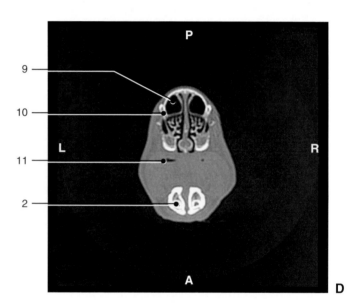

Figure 7-39, A-I
Type of animal: Rabbit
Type of study: CT head
Imaging plane: Transverse
Weight of animal: 4.1 kg
Gender: Female
Reproductive status: Intact
Age: Adult

1. External nare
2. Mandible
3. Mandibular incisor tooth
4. Nasal bone
5. Incisive bone
6. Nasoturbinates
7. Nasal septum
8. Maxillary incisor tooth
9. Frontal sinus
10. Frontal bone
11. Oral cavity
12. Nasopharynx
13. Vomer
14. Maxillary molar tooth
15. Masseter muscle

16. Mandibular molar tooth
17. Palatine bone
18. Ethmoturbinates
19. Sphenopalatine sinus
20. Zygomatic bone
21. Tympanic cavity
22. Tympanic bulla
23. Occipital bone
24. Parietal bone
25. Inner ear
26. Larynx
27. Ear canal
28. Occipital condyle
29. Atlas

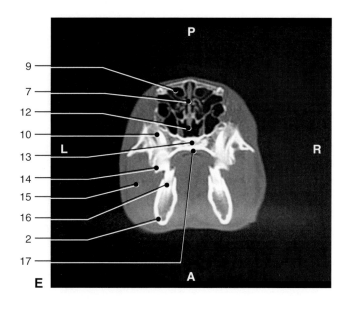

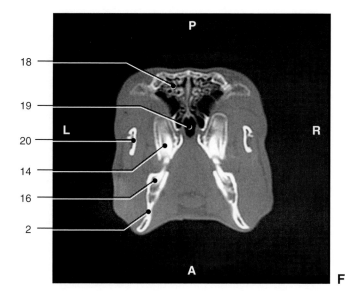

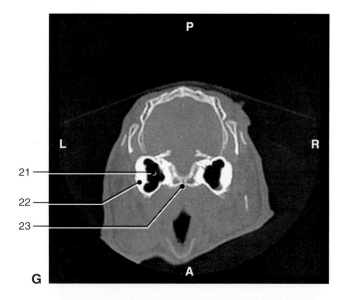

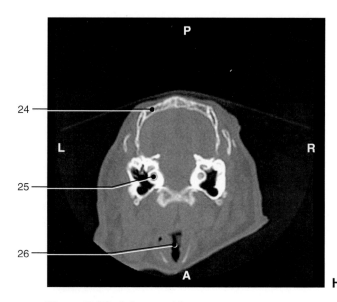

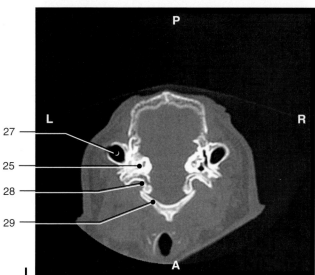

Figure 7-39, A-I—cont'd
Type of animal: Rabbit
Type of study: CT head
Imaging plane: Transverse
Weight of animal: 4.1 kg
Gender: Female
Reproductive status: Intact
Age: Adult

1. External nare
2. Mandible
3. Mandibular incisor tooth
4. Nasal bone
5. Incisive bone
6. Nasoturbinates
7. Nasal septum
8. Maxillary incisor tooth
9. Frontal sinus
10. Frontal bone
11. Oral cavity
12. Nasopharynx
13. Vomer
14. Maxillary molar tooth
15. Masseter muscle
16. Mandibular molar tooth
17. Palatine bone
18. Ethmoturbinates
19. Sphenopalatine sinus
20. Zygomatic bone
21. Tympanic cavity
22. Tympanic bulla
23. Occipital bone
24. Parietal bone
25. Inner ear
26. Larynx
27. Ear canal
28. Occipital condyle
29. Atlas

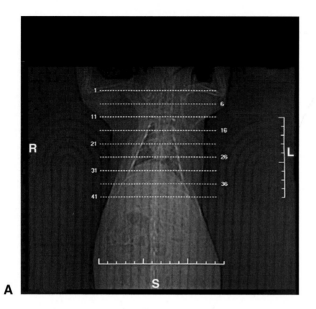

A

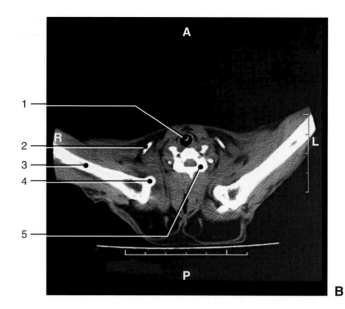

B

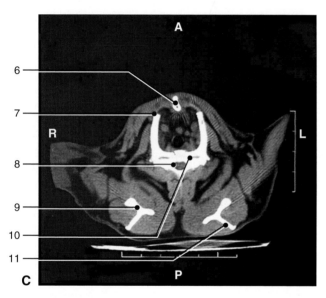

C

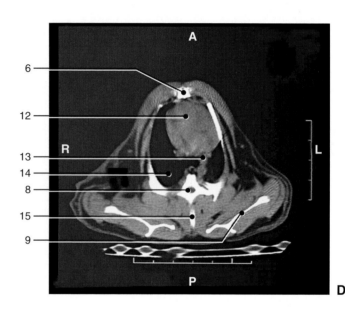

D

Figure 7-40, A-E

Type of animal: Rabbit
Type of study: CT thorax
Imaging plane: Transverse
Weight of Animal: 3.5 kg
Gender: Female
Reproductive status: Intact
Age: Adult

1. Trachea
2. Clavicle
3. Humerus
4. Humeral head
5. Cervical vertebra
6. Sternebra
7. Rib
8. Spinal canal of thoracic vertebra

9. Scapula
10. Thoracic vertebra
11. Spine of scapula
12. Heart
13. Aorta
14. Lung
15. Spinous process of thoracic vertebra
16. Pulmonary vasculature

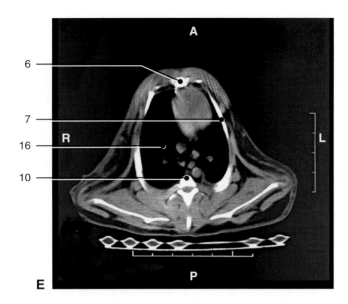

Figure 7-40, A-E—cont'd
Type of animal: Rabbit
Type of study: CT thorax
Imaging plane: Transverse
Weight of Animal: 3.5 kg
Gender: Female
Reproductive status: Intact
Age: Adult

1. Trachea
2. Clavicle
3. Humerus
4. Humeral head
5. Cervical vertebra
6. Sternebra
7. Rib
8. Spinal canal of thoracic vertebra
9. Scapula
10. Thoracic vertebra
11. Spine of scapula
12. Heart
13. Aorta
14. Lung
15. Spinous process of thoracic vertebra
16. Pulmonary vasculature

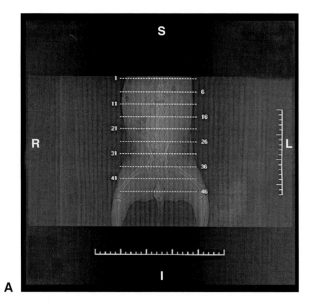

A

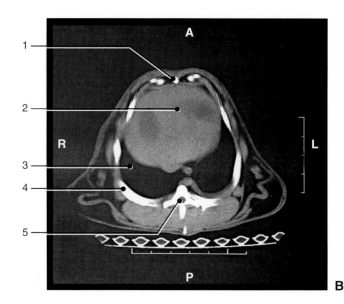

B

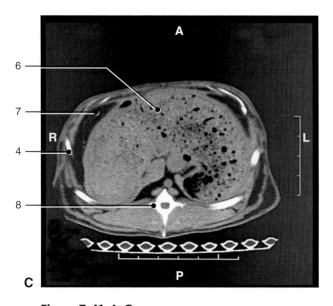

C

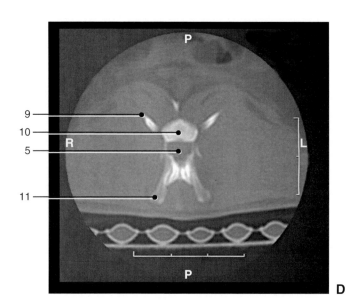

D

Figure 7-41, A-G

Type of animal: Rabbit
Type of study: CT abdomen
Imaging plane: Transverse
Weight of animal: 3.5 kg
Gender: Female
Reproductive status: Intact
Age: Adult

1. Sternebra
2. Liver
3. Lung
4. Rib
5. Spinal canal of thoracic vertebra
6. Stomach
7. Abdominal cavity
8. Thoracic vertebra
9. Transverse process of lumbar vertebra

10. Lumbar vertebra
11. Articular process of lumbar vertebra
12. Spinous process of lumbar vertebra
13. Sacrum
14. Ilium
15. Spinous process of sacral vertebra
16. Femoral head
17. Acetabulum
18. Caudal vertebra

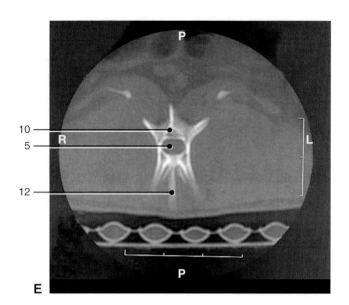

E

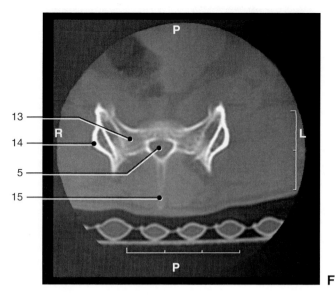

F

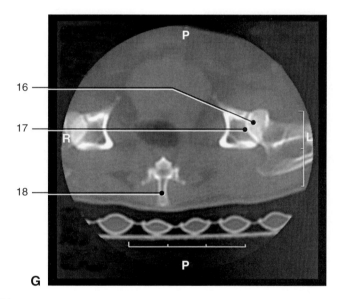

G

Figure 7-41, A-G—cont'd

Type of animal: Rabbit
Type of study: CT abdomen
Imaging plane: Transverse
Weight of animal: 3.5 kg
Gender: Female
Reproductive status: Intact
Age: Adult

1. Sternebra
2. Liver
3. Lung
4. Rib
5. Spinal canal of thoracic vertebra
6. Stomach
7. Abdominal cavity
8. Thoracic vertebra
9. Transverse process of lumbar vertebra

10. Lumbar vertebra
11. Articular process of lumbar vertebra
12. Spinous process of lumbar vertebra
13. Sacrum
14. Ilium
15. Spinous process of sacral vertebra
16. Femoral head
17. Acetabulum
18. Caudal vertebra

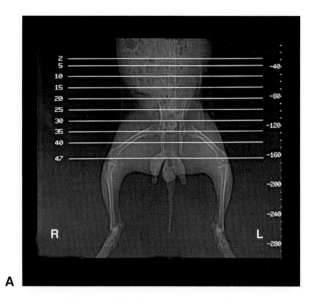

A

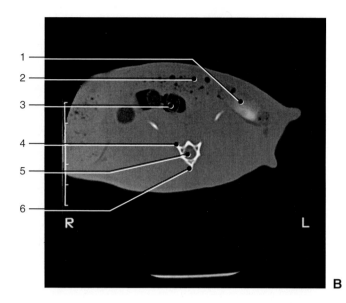

B

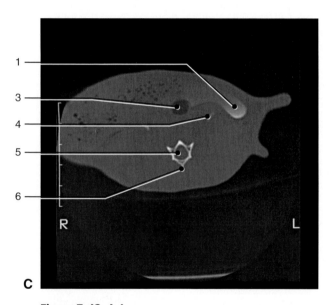

C

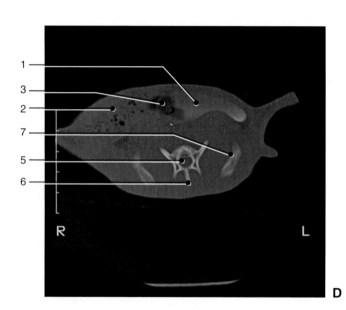

D

Figure 7-42, A-I
Type of animal: Rabbit
Type of study: CT pelvis
Imaging plane: Transverse
Weight of animal: 3.5 kg
Gender: Female
Reproductive status: Intact
Age: Adult

1. Urinary bladder
2. Cecum
3. Colon
4. Transverse process of lumbar vertebra
5. Spinal canal of lumbar vertebra
6. Spinous process of lumbar vertebra
7. Ilium
8. Caudal end plate of 7th lumbar vertebra
9. Articular process of lumbar vertebra
10. Sacroiliac joint

11. Spinous process of sacral vertebra
12. Sacral vertebra
13. Spinal canal of sacral vertebra
14. Femur
15. Femoral neck
16. Femoral head
17. Acetabulum
18. Lunate surface of acetabulum
19. Caudal vertebra

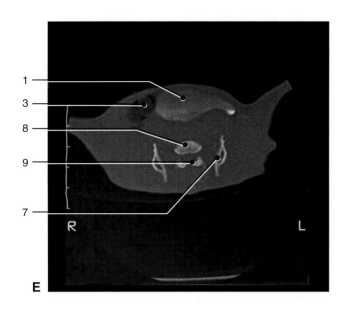

E

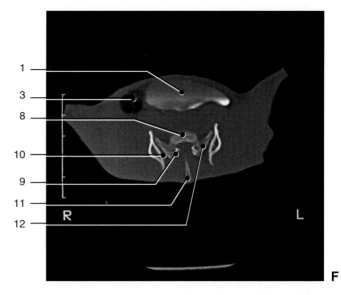

F

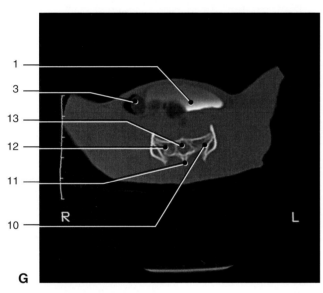

G

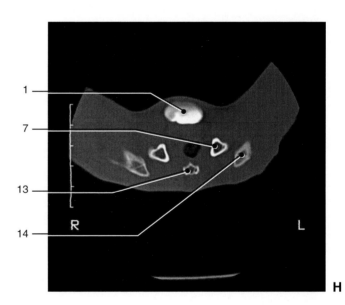

H

Figure 7-42, A-I—cont'd
Type of animal: Rabbit
Type of study: CT pelvis
Imaging plane: Transverse
Weight of animal: 3.5 kg
Gender: Female
Reproductive status: Intact
Age: Adult

1. Urinary bladder
2. Cecum
3. Colon
4. Transverse process of lumbar vertebra
5. Spinal canal of lumbar vertebra
6. Spinous process of lumbar vertebra
7. Ilium
8. Caudal end plate of 7th lumbar vertebra
9. Articular process of lumbar vertebra
10. Sacroiliac joint

11. Spinous process of sacral vertebra
12. Sacral vertebra
13. Spinal canal of sacral vertebra
14. Femur
15. Femoral neck
16. Femoral head
17. Acetabulum
18. Lunate surface of acetabulum
19. Caudal vertebra

Figure 7-42, A-I—cont'd
Type of animal: Rabbit
Type of study: CT pelvis
Imaging plane: Transverse
Weight of animal: 3.5 kg
Gender: Female
Reproductive status: Intact
Age: Adult

1. Urinary bladder
2. Cecum
3. Colon
4. Transverse process of lumbar vertebra
5. Spinal canal of lumbar vertebra
6. Spinous process of lumbar vertebra
7. Ilium
8. Caudal end plate of 7th lumbar vertebra
9. Articular process of lumbar vertebra
10. Sacroiliac joint
11. Spinous process of sacral vertebra
12. Sacral vertebra
13. Spinal canal of sacral vertebra
14. Femur
15. Femoral neck
16. Femoral head
17. Acetabulum
18. Lunate surface of acetabulum
19. Caudal vertebra

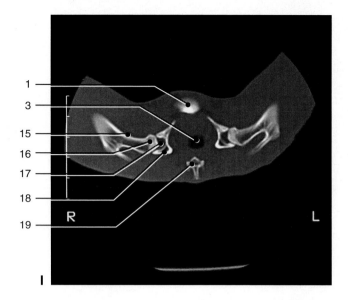

CHAPTER 8

Domestic Ferret *(Mustela putorius)*

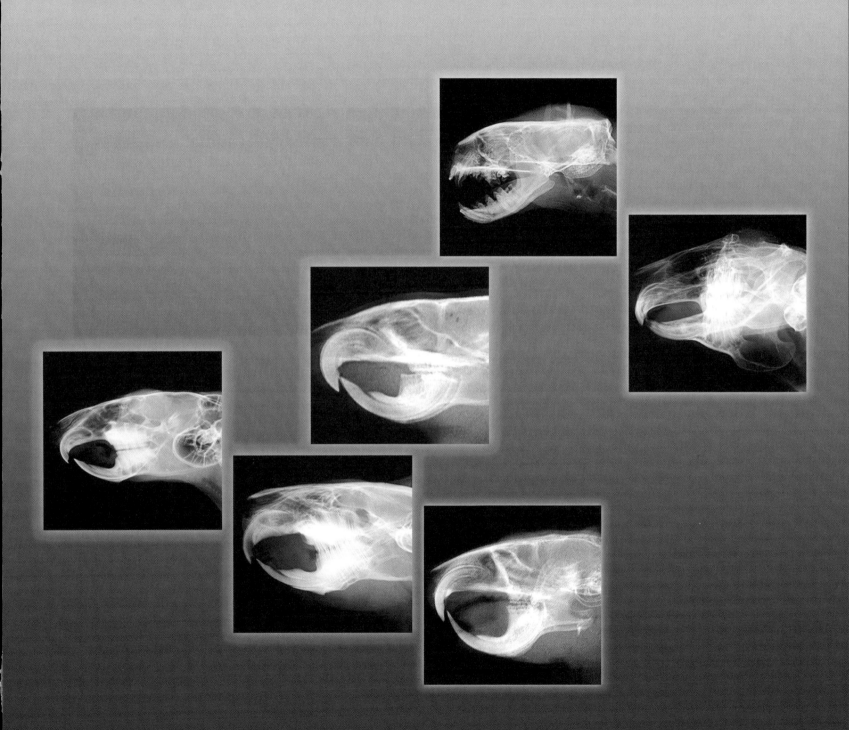

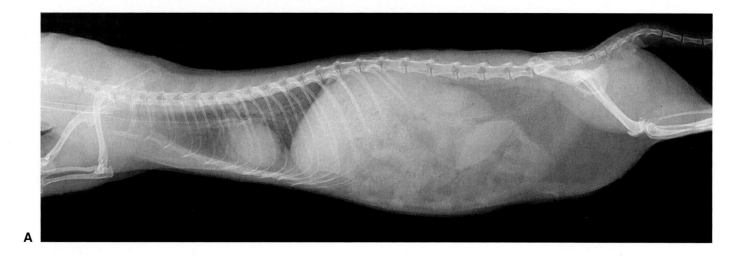

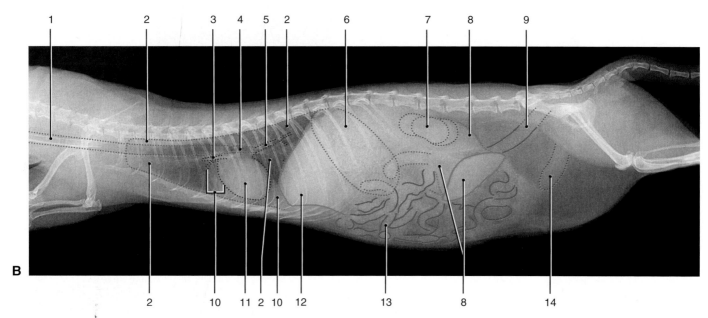

Figure 8-1, A and B
Type of animal: Ferret
Type of study: Viscera of thorax and abdomen
Projection: Laterolateral (right lateral recumbency)
Weight of animal: 900 g
Gender: Female
Reproductive status: Spayed
Age: 1 year

1. Trachea (endotracheal tube within lumen)
2. Lung
3. Pulmonary vasculature
4. Bronchus
5. Pulmonary vein
6. Stomach
7. Kidney
8. Spleen
9. Colon
10. Intrathoracic adipose tissue
11. Heart
12. Liver
13. Small intestine
14. Urinary bladder

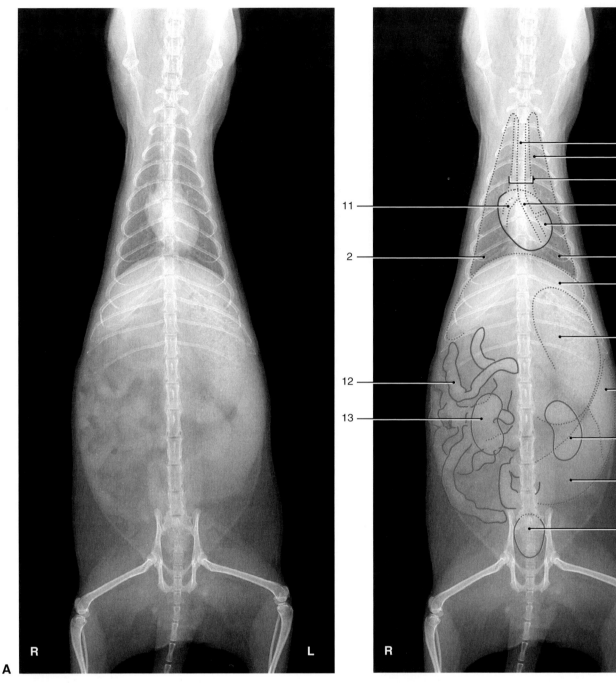

Figure 8-2, A
Type of animal: Ferret
Type of study: Viscera of thorax
    and abdomen
Projection: Ventrodorsal
Weight of animal: 900 g
Gender: Female
Reproductive status: Spayed
Age: 1 year

Figure 8-2, B
Type of animal: Ferret
Type of study: Viscera of thorax and abdomen
Projection: Ventrodorsal
Weight of animal: 900 g
Gender: Female
Reproductive status: Spayed
Age: 1 year

1. Trachea (endotracheal tube within lumen)
2. Lung
3. Cranial mediastinum
4. Left primary bronchus
5. Heart
6. Liver
7. Stomach
8. Spleen
9. Left kidney
10. Urinary bladder
11. Right primary bronchus
12. Small intestine
13. Right kidney

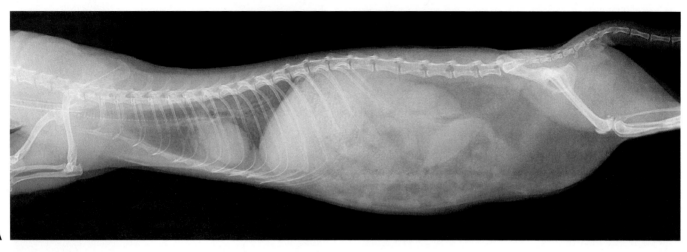

Figure 8-3, A
Type of animal: Ferret
Type of study: Whole body skeleton
Projection: Laterolateral (right lateral recumbency)
Weight of animal: 900 g
Gender: Female
Reproductive status: Spayed
Age: 1 year

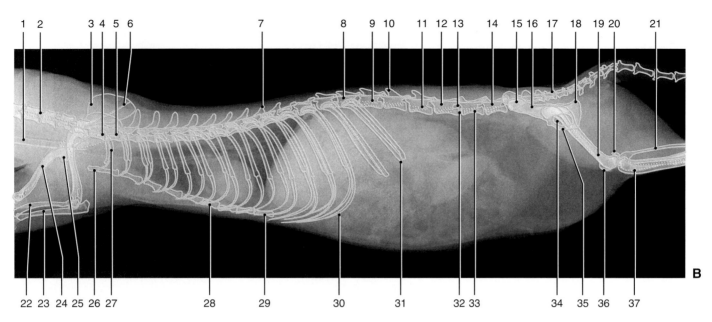

Figure 8-3, B
Type of animal: Ferret
Type of study: Whole body skeleton
Projection: Laterolateral (right lateral recumbency)
Weight of animal: 900 g
Gender: Female
Reproductive status: Spayed
Age: 1 year

1. Trachea (endotracheal tube within lumen)
2. Cervical intervertebral space
3. Scapula
4. 7th cervical vertebra
5. 1st thoracic vertebra
6. Spine of scapula
7. Spinous process of thoracic vertebra
8. 14th thoracic vertebra
9. 1st lumbar vertebra
10. Spinous process of lumbar vertebra
11. Ventral margin of spinal canal
12. Spinal canal
13. Lumbar intervertebral foramen
14. 6th lumbar vertebra
15. Sacrum
16. Ilium
17. 1st caudal vertebra
18. Ischium
19. Femur
20. Fabella
21. Fibula
22. Radius
23. Ulna
24. Humerus
25. Humeral head
26. Manubrium of sternum
27. 1st rib
28. Sternebra
29. Xyphoid process
30. Costal cartilage
31. 14th rib
32. Lumbar intervertebral space
33. Transverse process of lumbar vertebra
34. Obturator foramen
35. Pubis
36. Patella
37. Tibia

Figure 8-4, A
Type of animal: Ferret
Type of study: Whole body skeleton
Projection: Ventrodorsal
Weight of animal: 900 g
Gender: Female
Reproductive status: Spayed
Age: 1 year

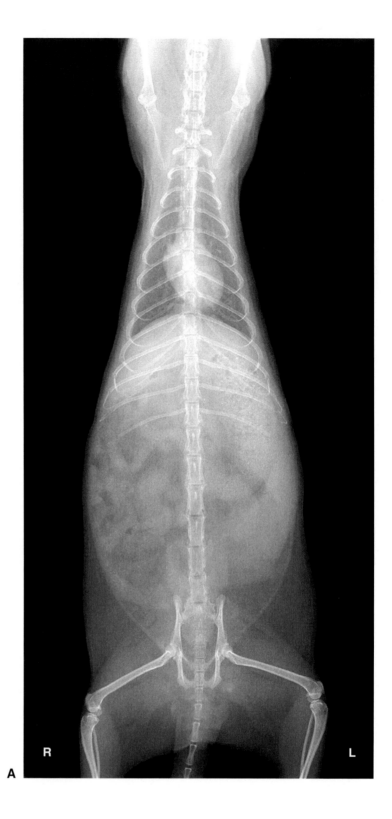

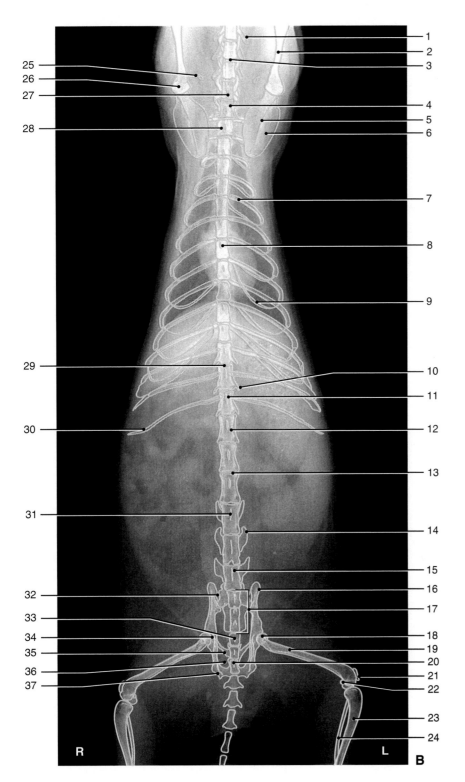

Figure 8-4, B
Type of animal: Ferret
Type of study: Whole body skeleton
Projection: Ventrodorsal
Weight of animal: 900 g
Gender: Female
Reproductive status: Spayed
Age: 1 year

1. Transverse process of cervical vertebra
2. Humerus
3. Cervical intervertebral space
4. 7th cervical vertebra
5. Spine of scapula
6. Scapula
7. 5th rib
8. Spinous process of thoracic vertebra
9. Costal cartilage
10. Transverse process of thoracic vertebra
11. 14th thoracic vertebra
12. 1st lumbar vertebra
13. Lumbar intervertebral space
14. Transverse process of lumbar vertebra
15. 6th lumbar vertebra
16. Ilium
17. Sacrum
18. Femoral head
19. Femur
20. Spinous process of caudal vertebra
21. Patella
22. Fabella
23. Tibia
24. Fibula
25. Clavicle
26. Humeral head
27. Spinous process of cervical vertebra
28. 1st thoracic vertebra
29. Thoracic intervertebral space
30. 14th rib
31. Spinous process of lumbar vertebra
32. Sacroiliac joint
33. 1st caudal vertebra
34. Acetabulum
35. Pubis
36. Obturator foramen
37. Ischium

Figure 8-5, A
Type of animal: Ferret
Type of study: Head
Projection: Laterolateral
 (right lateral recumbency)
Weight of animal: 1.2 kg
Gender: Male
Reproductive status: Neutered
Age: Adult

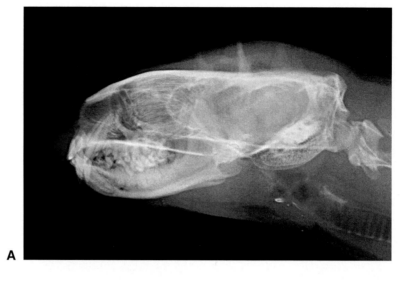

A

Figure 8-5, B
Type of animal: Ferret
Type of study: Head
Projection: Laterolateral
 (right lateral recumbency)
Weight of animal: 1.2 kg
Gender: Male
Reproductive status: Neutered
Age: Adult

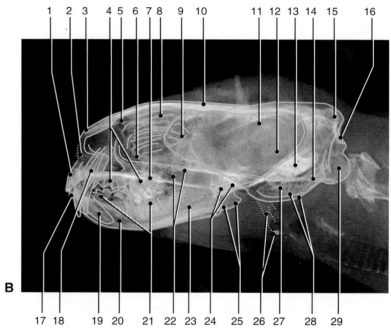

B

1. Maxillary incisor tooth
2. Incisive bone
3. Nasal bone
4. Maxillary premolar and
   molar teeth
5. Nasal cavity
6. Maxilla
7. Hard palate
8. Nasoturbinates
9. Ethmoturbinates
10. Frontal bone
11. Parietal bone
12. Temporal bone
13. Petrous part of temporal bone
14. Basal part of occipital bone
15. Occipital protuberance
16. Occipital bone
17. Mandibular incisor tooth
18. Maxillary canine tooth
19. Mandibular canine tooth
20. Mental foramen
21. Mandibular premolar
    and molar teeth
22. Coronoid processes of mandible
23. Mandibular foramen
24. Condylar processes of mandible
25. Angular processes of mandible
26. Hyoid bones
27. Tympanic cavity
28. Tympanic bullae
29. Occipital condyle

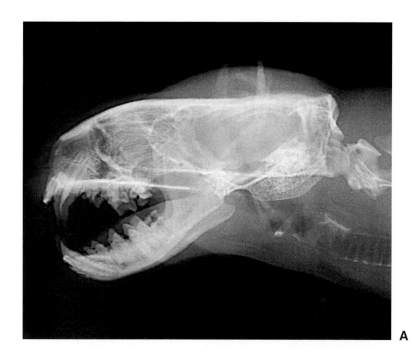

Figure 8-6, A
Type of animal: Ferret
Type of study: Head with open mouth
Projection: Laterolateral
    (right lateral recumbency)
Weight of animal: 1.2 kg
Gender: Male
Reproductive status: Neutered
Age: Adult

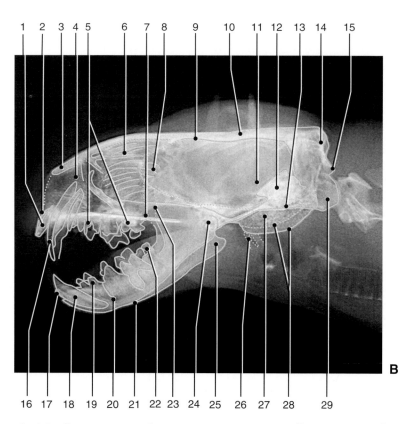

Figure 8-6, B
Type of animal: Ferret
Type of study: Head with open mouth
Projection: Laterolateral
    (right lateral recumbency)
Weight of animal: 1.2 kg
Gender: Male
Reproductive status: Neutered
Age: Adult

1. Maxillary incisor tooth
2. Incisive bone
3. Nasal bone
4. Nasal cavity
5. Maxillary premolar and molar teeth
6. Nasoturbinates
7. Palatine bone
8. Ethmoturbinates
9. Frontal bone
10. Parietal bone
11. Temporal bone
12. Petrous part of temporal bone
13. Basal part of occipital bone
14. External occipital protuberance
15. Occipital bone
16. Maxillary canine tooth
17. Mandibular incisor tooth
18. Mandibular canine tooth
19. Mandibular premolar tooth
20. Mental foramen
21. Mandible
22. Mandibular molar tooth
23. Coronoid process of mandible
24. Condylar process of mandible
25. Angular process of mandible
26. Hyoid bones
27. Tympanic cavity
28. Tympanic bullae
29. Occipital condyle

Figure 8-7, A
Type of animal: Ferret
Type of study: Head
Projection: Dorsoventral
Weight of animal: 1.2 kg
Gender: Male
Reproductive status: Neutered
Age: Adult

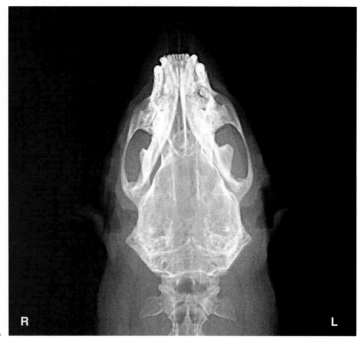

A

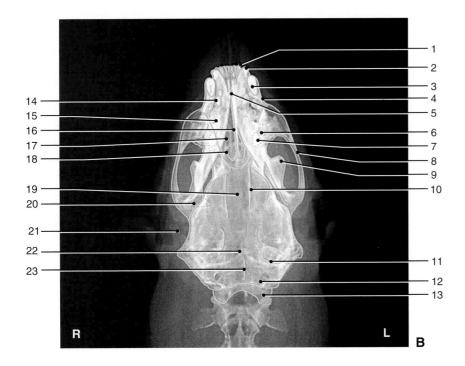

Figure 8-7, B
Type of animal: Ferret
Type of study: Head
Projection: Dorsoventral
Weight of animal: 1.2 kg
Gender: Male
Reproductive status: Neutered
Age: Adult

1. Incisor tooth
2. Mandibular canine tooth
3. Maxillary canine tooth
4. Maxilla
5. Mandibular symphysis
6. Frontal bone
7. Molar tooth
8. Zygomatic bone
9. Coronoid process
   of mandible
10. Pterygoid bone
11. Tympanic bulla
12. Occipital bone
13. Occipital condyle
14. Premolar tooth
15. Mandible
16. Vomer
17. Nasal cavity
18. Ethmoturbinates
19. Presphenoidal bone
20. Temporomandibular joint
21. Ear canal
22. Basisphenoidal bone
23. Sagittal crest

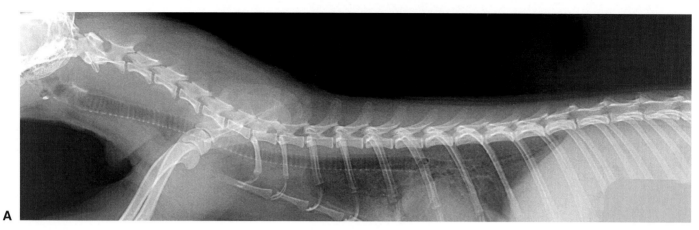

Figure 8-8, A
Type of animal: Ferret
Type of study: Cervical and thoracic vertebral column
Projection: Laterolateral (right lateral recumbency)
Weight of animal: 1.2 kg
Gender: Male
Reproductive status: Neutered
Age: Adult

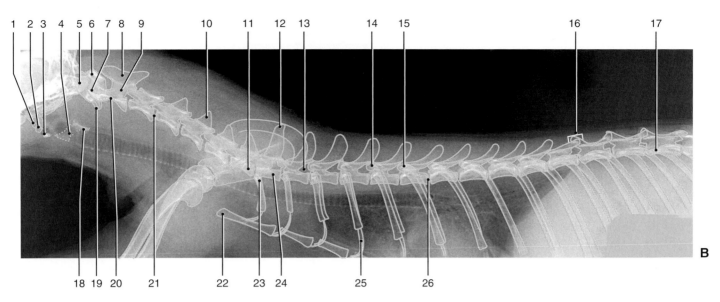

Figure 8-8, B
Type of animal: Ferret
Type of study: Cervical and thoracic vertebral column
Projection: Laterolateral (right lateral recumbency)
Weight of animal: 1.2 kg
Gender: Male
Reproductive status: Neutered
Age: Adult

1. Epihyoid bone
2. Ceratohyoid bone
3. Basihyoid bone
4. Thyroid cartilage
5. Occipital condyle
6. Dorsal tubercle of atlas
7. Dens of axis
8. Spinous process of axis
9. Spinal canal
10. Spinous process of cervical vertebra
11. 7th cervical vertebra
12. Spinous process of thoracic vertebra
13. Thoracic intervertebral foramen
14. Transverse process of thoracic vertebra
15. Head of rib
16. Articular processes of thoracic vertebrae
17. 14th thoracic vertebra
18. Cricoid cartilage
19. Transverse process of atlas
20. Transverse process of axis
21. Cervical intervertebral space
22. Manubrium of sternum
23. 1st rib
24. 1st thoracic vertebra
25. Costal cartilage
26. Thoracic intervertebral space

Figure 8-9, A
Type of animal: Ferret
Type of study: Cervical
    and thoracic vertebral column
Projection: Ventrodorsal
Weight of animal: 1.2 kg
Gender: Male
Reproductive status: Neutered
Age: Adult

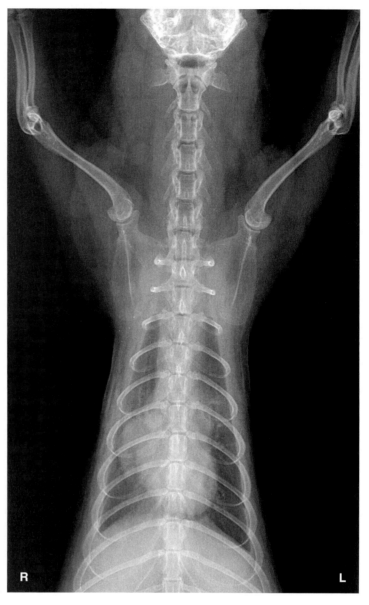

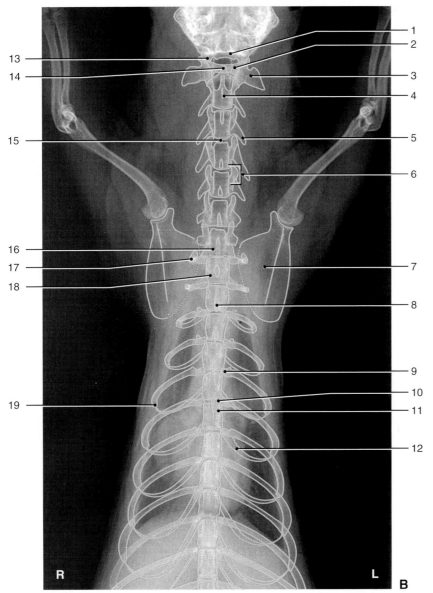

Figure 8-9, B
Type of animal: Ferret
Type of study: Cervical
　and thoracic vertebral column
Projection: Ventrodorsal
Weight of animal: 1.2 kg
Gender: Male
Reproductive status: Neutered
Age: Adult

1. Occipital bone
2. Atlas
3. Transverse process of atlas
4. Spinous process of axis
5. Transverse process of cervical vertebra
6. Articular processes of cervical vertebrae
7. Scapula
8. Spinous process of thoracic vertebra
9. Head of rib
10. Thoracic intervertebral space
11. Articular process of thoracic vertebra
12. Costal cartilage
13. Occipital condyle
14. Dens of axis
15. Cervical intervertebral space
16. 7th cervical vertebra
17. 1st rib
18. 1st thoracic vertebra
19. Costochondral joint

Figure 8-10, A
Type of animal: Ferret
Type of study: Lumbar, sacral,
    and caudal vertebral column
Projection: Laterolateral
    (right lateral recumbency)
Weight of animal: 1.2 kg
Gender: Male
Reproductive status: Neutered
Age: Adult

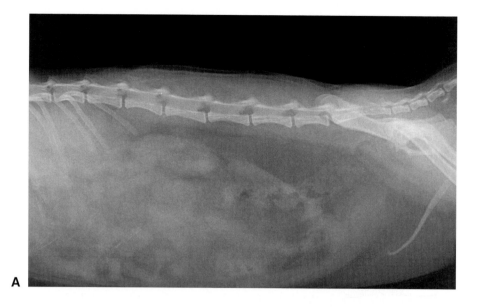

A

Figure 8-10, B
Type of animal: Ferret
Type of study: Lumbar, sacral,
    and caudal vertebral column
Projection: Laterolateral
    (right lateral recumbency)
Weight of animal: 1.2 kg
Gender: Male
Reproductive status: Neutered
Age: Adult

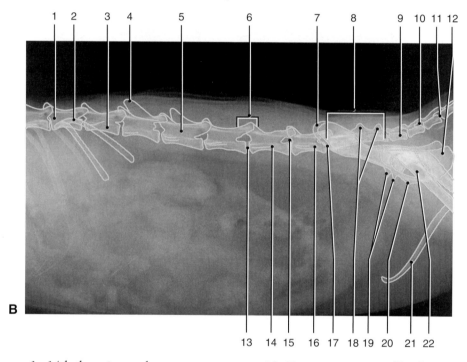

B

1. 14th thoracic vertebra
2. Rib
3. 1st lumbar vertebra
4. Spinous process of lumbar vertebra
5. Spinal canal
6. Articular processes of lumbar vertebrae
7. Ilium
8. Sacrum
9. 1st caudal vertebra
10. Caudal intervertebral foramen
11. Caudal intervertebral space
12. Ischium
13. Lumbar intervertebral space
14. Transverse process of lumbar vertebra
15. Lumbar intervertebral foramen
16. 6th lumbar vertebra
17. Lumbosacral intervertebral space
18. Spinous processes of sacral vertebrae
19. Iliopubic eminence
20. Pubis
21. Os penis
22. Obturator foramen

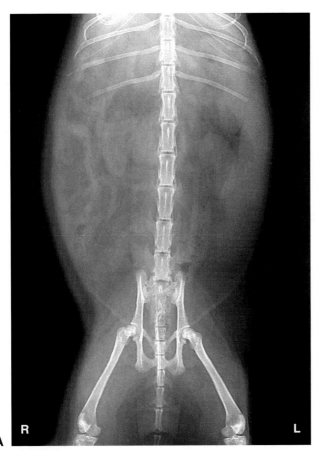

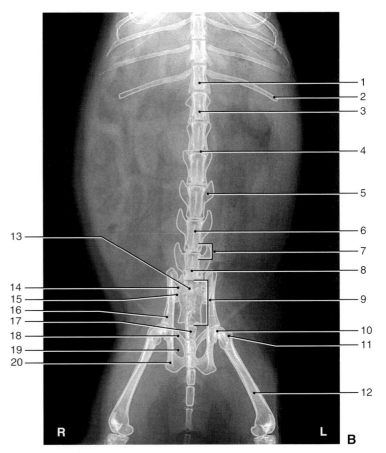

Figure 8-11, A
Type of animal: Ferret
Type of study: Lumbar, sacral,
  and caudal vertebral column
Projection: Ventrodorsal
Weight of animal: 1.2 kg
Gender: Male
Reproductive status: Neutered
Age: Adult

Figure 8-11, B
Type of animal: Ferret
Type of study: Lumbar, sacral,
  and caudal vertebral column
Projection: Ventrodorsal
Weight of animal: 1.2 kg
Gender: Male
Reproductive status: Neutered
Age: Adult

1. 14th thoracic vertebra
2. 14th rib
3. 1st lumbar vertebra
4. Lumbar intervertebral space
5. Transverse process of lumbar vertebra
6. Spinous process of lumbar vertebra
7. Articular processes of lumbar vertebrae
8. 6th lumbar vertebra
9. Sacrum
10. Femoral head
11. Greater trochanter of femur
12. Femur
13. Spinous process of sacral vertebra
14. Sacral foramen
15. Sacroiliac joint
16. Ilium
17. 1st caudal vertebra
18. Pubis
19. Obturator foramen
20. Ischium

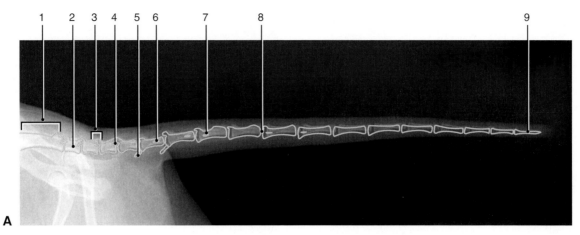

Figure 8-12, A
Type of animal: Ferret
Type of study: Caudal vertebral column
Projection: Laterolateral
Weight of animal: 1.2 kg
Gender: Male
Reproductive status: Neutered
Age: Adult

1. Sacrum
2. 1st caudal vertebra
3. Articular processes of caudal vertebrae
4. Caudal intervertebral foramen
5. Hemal arch of caudal vertebra
6. Caudal articular process
7. Transverse process of caudal vertebra
8. Caudal intervertebral space
9. Last caudal vertebra

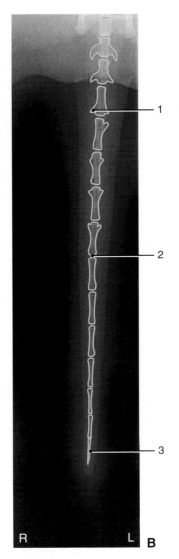

Figure 8-12, B
Type of animal: Ferret
Type of study: Caudal vertebral column
Projection: Ventrodorsal
Weight of animal: 1.2 kg
Gender: Male
Reproductive status: Neutered
Age: Adult

1. Caudal articular process
2. Caudal intervertebral space
3. Last caudal vertebra

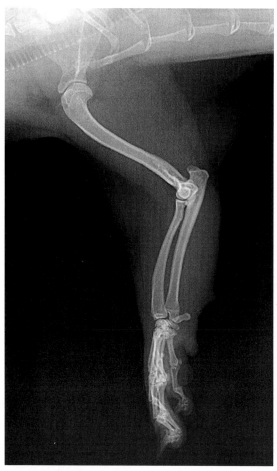

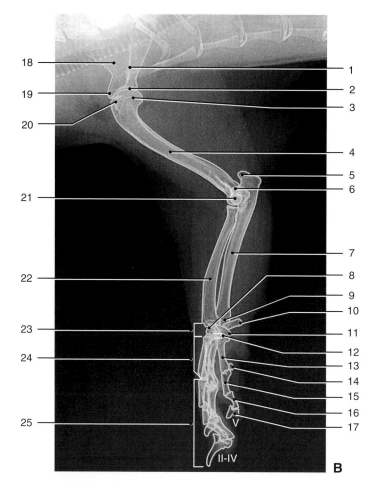

Figure 8-13, A
Type of animal: Ferret
Type of study: Thoracic limb
Projection: Mediolateral
Weight of animal: 1.2 kg
Gender: Male
Reproductive status: Neutered
Age: Adult

Figure 8-13, B
Type of animal: Ferret
Type of study: Thoracic limb
Projection: Mediolateral
Weight of animal: 1.2 kg
Gender: Male
Reproductive status: Neutered
Age: Adult

1. Spine of scapula
2. Scapulohumeral joint space
3. Humeral head
4. Humerus
5. Olecranon of ulna
6. Anconeal process of olecranon
7. Ulna
8. Radial carpal bone
9. Styloid process of ulna
10. Accessory carpal bone
11. Ulnar carpal bone
12. Carpal bones I, II, III, and IV
13. Metacarpal bone V
14. Proximal sesamoid bone
15. Proximal phalanx of digit V
16. Middle phalanx of digit V
17. Distal phalanx of digit V
18. Scapula
19. Supraglenoid tubercle
20. Greater tubercle of humerus
21. Humeral condyle
22. Radius
23. Carpal bones
24. Metacarpal bones
25. Phalanges

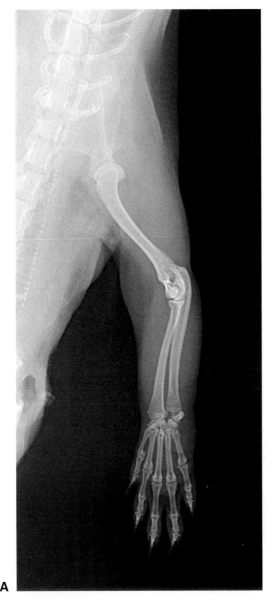

Figure 8-14, A
Type of animal: Ferret
Type of study: Thoracic limb
Projection: Ventrodorsal
Weight of animal: 1.2 kg
Gender: Male
Reproductive status: Neutered
Age: Adult

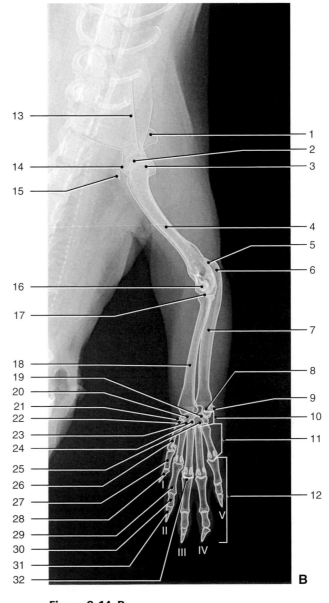

Figure 8-14, B
Type of animal: Ferret
Type of study: Thoracic limb
Projection: Ventrodorsal
Weight of animal: 1.2 kg
Gender: Male
Reproductive status: Neutered
Age: Adult

1. Acromion
2. Scapulohumeral joint space
3. Humeral head
4. Humerus
5. Humeral epicondyle
6. Olecranon of ulna
7. Ulna
8. Styloid process of ulna
9. Accessory carpal bone
10. Carpal bones
11. Metacarpal bones
12. Phalanges
13. Spine of scapula
14. Supraglenoid tubercle
15. Clavicle
16. Humeral condyle

17. Humeroradial joint space
18. Radius
19. Ulnar carpal bone
20. Radial carpal bone
21. Palmar sesamoid bone
22. Carpal bone I
23. Carpal bone II
24. Carpal bone III
25. Carpal bone IV
26. Metacarpal bone I
27. Proximal phalanx of digit I
28. Distal phalanx of digit I
29. Proximal phalanx of digit II
30. Middle phalanx of digit II
31. Distal phalanx of digit II
32. Proximal sesamoid bones

Figure 8-15, A
Type of animal: Ferret
Type of study: Elbow joint
Projection: Mediolateral
Weight of animal: 1.2 kg
Gender: Male
Reproductive status: Neutered
Age: Adult

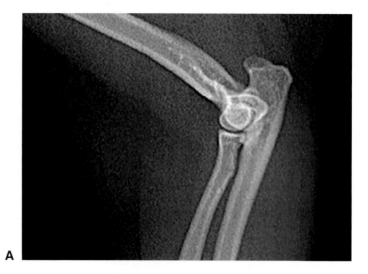

A

Figure 8-15, B
Type of animal: Ferret
Type of study: Elbow joint
Projection: Mediolateral
Weight of animal: 1.2 kg
Gender: Male
Reproductive status: Neutered
Age: Adult

1. Olecranon of ulna
2. Anconeal process of olecranon
3. Ulna
4. Humerus
5. Humeral condyle
6. Radius

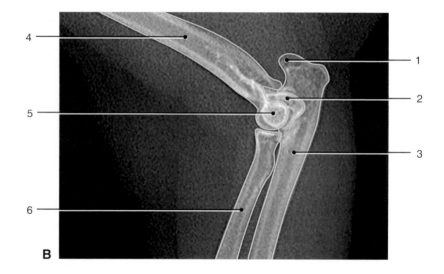

B

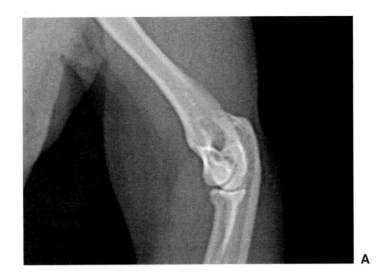

Figure 8-16, A
Type of animal: Ferret
Type of study: Elbow joint
Projection: Caudocranial
Weight of animal: 1.2 kg
Gender: Male
Reproductive status: Neutered
Age: Adult

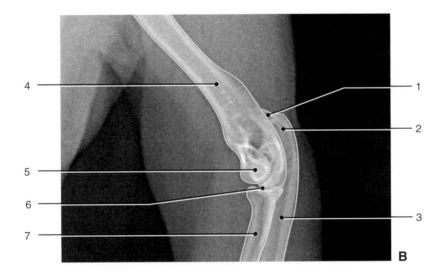

Figure 8-16, B
Type of animal: Ferret
Type of study: Elbow joint
Projection: Caudocranial
Weight of animal: 1.2 kg
Gender: Male
Reproductive status: Neutered
Age: Adult

1. Humeral epicondyle
2. Olecranon of ulna
3. Ulna
4. Humerus
5. Humeral condyle
6. Humeroradial joint space
7. Radius

Figure 8-17, A
Type of animal: Ferret
Type of study: Distal thoracic limb
Projection: Mediolateral
Weight of animal: 1.2 kg
Gender: Male
Reproductive status: Neutered
Age: Adult

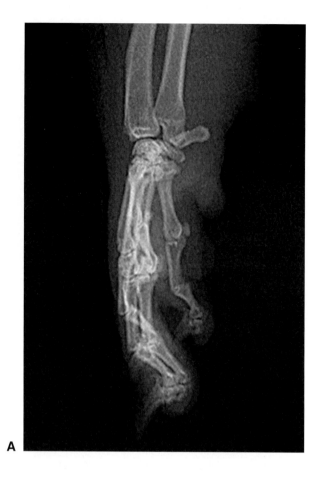

A

Figure 8-17, B
Type of animal: Ferret
Type of study: Distal thoracic limb
Projection: Mediolateral
Weight of animal: 1.2 kg
Gender: Male
Reproductive status: Neutered
Age: Adult

1. Radial carpal bone
2. Styloid process of ulna
3. Accessory carpal bone
4. Ulnar carpal bone
5. Carpal bones I, II, III, and IV
6. Metacarpal bone V
7. Proximal sesamoid bone
8. Proximal phalanx of digit V
9. Middle phalanx of digit V
10. Distal phalanx of digit V
11. Radius
12. Ulna
13. Carpal bones
14. Metacarpal bones
15. Phalanges

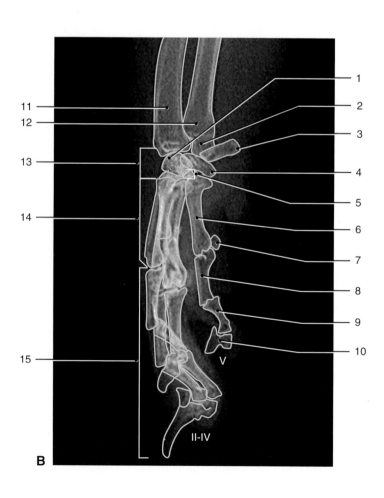

B

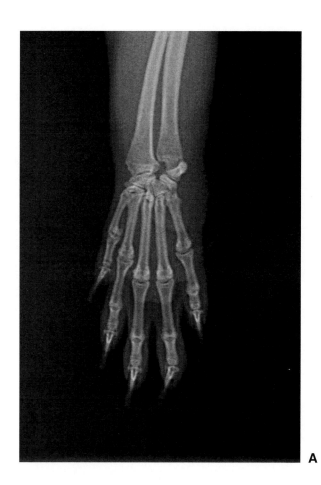

A

Figure 8-18, A
Type of animal: Ferret
Type of study: Distal thoracic limb
Projection: Dorsopalmar
Weight of animal: 1.2 kg
Gender: Male
Reproductive status: Neutered
Age: Adult

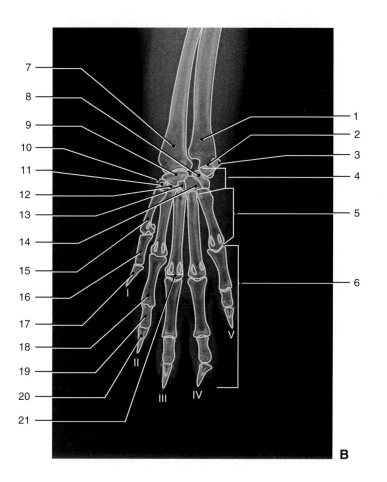

B

Figure 8-18, B
Type of animal: Ferret
Type of study: Distal thoracic limb
Projection: Dorsopalmar
Weight of animal: 1.2 kg
Gender: Male
Reproductive status: Neutered
Age: Adult

1. Ulna
2. Styloid process of ulna
3. Accessory carpal bone
4. Carpal bones
5. Metacarpal bones
6. Phalanges
7. Radius
8. Ulnar carpal bone
9. Radial carpal bone
10. Palmar sesamoid bone
11. Carpal bone I
12. Carpal bone II
13. Carpal bone III
14. Carpal bone IV
15. Metacarpal bone I
16. Proximal phalanx of digit I
17. Distal phalanx of digit I
18. Proximal phalanx of digit II
19. Middle phalanx of digit II
20. Distal phalanx of digit II
21. Proximal sesamoid bones

Figure 8-19, A
Type of animal: Ferret
Type of study: Pelvis
Projection: Laterolateral
   (right lateral recumbency)
Weight of animal: 1.2 kg
Gender: Male
Reproductive status: Neutered
Age: Adult

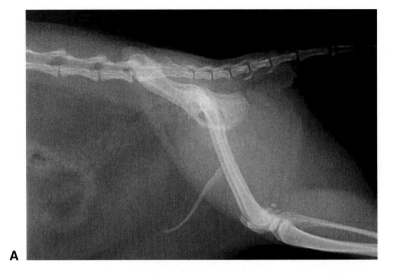

Figure 8-19, B
Type of animal: Ferret
Type of study: Pelvis
Projection: Laterolatera
   (right lateral recumbency)
Weight of animal: 1.2 kg
Gender: Male
Reproductive status: Neutered
Age: Adult

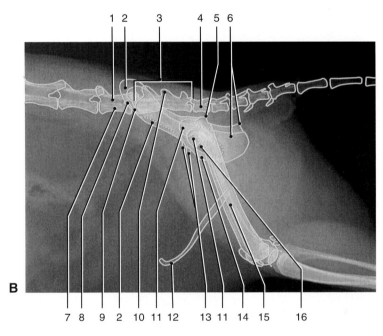

1. Spinal canal
2. Ilium
3. Sacrum
4. 1st caudal vertebra
5. Greater trochanter of femur
6. Ischia
7. 6th lumbar vertebra
8. Lumbosacral intervertebral foramen
9. Lumbosacral intervertebral space
10. Spinous process of sacral vertebra
11. Femoral head
12. Os penis
13. Iliopubic eminences
14. Pubis
15. Femur
16. Obturator foramen

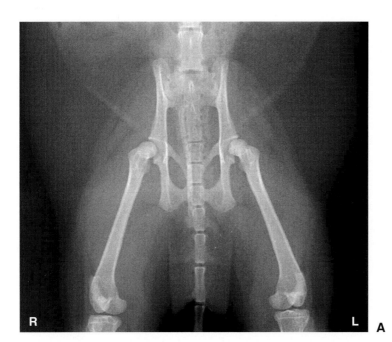

Figure 8-20, A
Type of animal: Ferret
Type of study: Pelvis
Projection: Ventrodorsal
Weight of animal: 1.2 kg
Gender: Male
Reproductive status: Neutered
Age: Adult

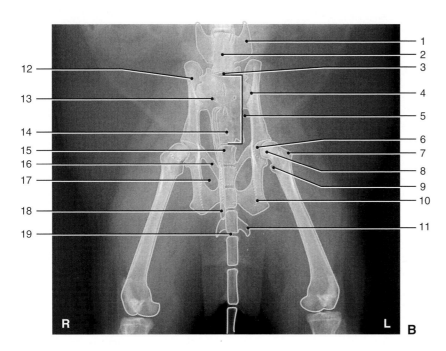

Figure 8-20, B
Type of animal: Ferret
Type of study: Pelvis
Projection: Ventrodorsal
Weight of animal: 1.2 kg
Gender: Male
Reproductive status: Neutered
Age: Adult

1. Transverse process of lumbar vertebra
2. 6th lumbar vertebra
3. Lumbosacral intervertebral space
4. Sacroiliac joint
5. Sacrum
6. Acetabulum
7. Greater trochanter of femur
8. Femoral head
9. Lesser trochanter of femur
10. Ischium
11. Transverse process of caudal vertebra
12. Ilium
13. Sacral foramen
14. Spinous process of sacral vertebra
15. 1st caudal vertebra
16. Pubis
17. Obturator foramen
18. Os penis
19. Caudal intervertebral space

Figure 8-21, A
Type of animal: Ferret
Type of study: Pelvic limb
Projection: Mediolateral
Weight of animal: 1.2 kg
Gender: Male
Reproductive status: Neutered
Age: Adult

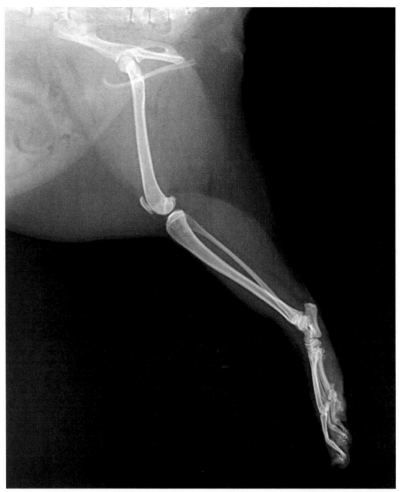

A

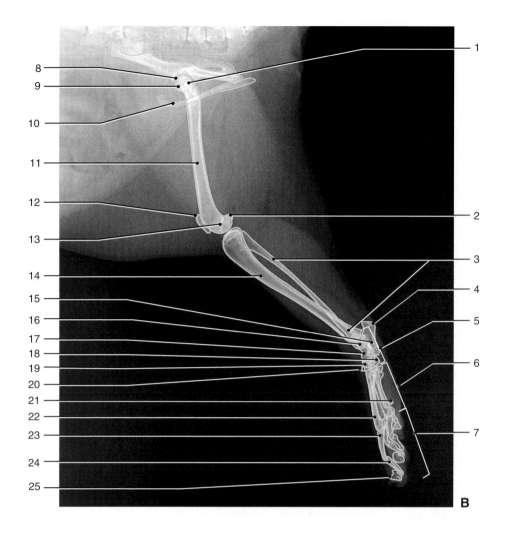

Figure 8-21, B
Type of animal: Ferret
Type of study: Pelvic limb
Projection: Mediolateral
Weight of animal: 1.2 kg
Gender: Male
Reproductive status: Neutered
Age: Adult

1. Greater trochanter of femur
2. Fabella
3. Fibula
4. Calcaneal tuber
5. Tarsal bones
6. Metatarsal bones
7. Phalanges
8. Acetabulum
9. Femoral head
10. Os penis
11. Femur
12. Patella
13. Femoral condyle
14. Tibia
15. Talus
16. Trochlea of talus
17. Calcaneus
18. Tarsal bone IV
19. Central tarsal bone
20. Tarsal bones I, II, and III
21. Proximal sesamoid bone
22. Metatarsal bone
23. Proximal phalanx
24. Middle phalanx
25. Distal phalanx

Figure 8-22, A
Type of animal: Ferret
Type of study: Pelvic limb
Projection: Ventrodorsal
Weight of animal: 1.2 kg
Gender: Male
Reproductive status: Neutered
Age: Adult

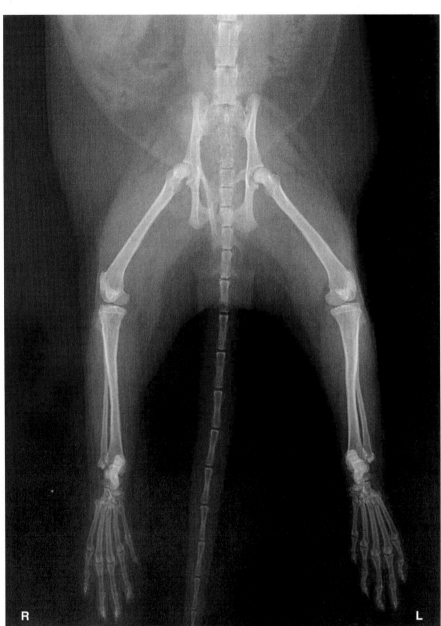

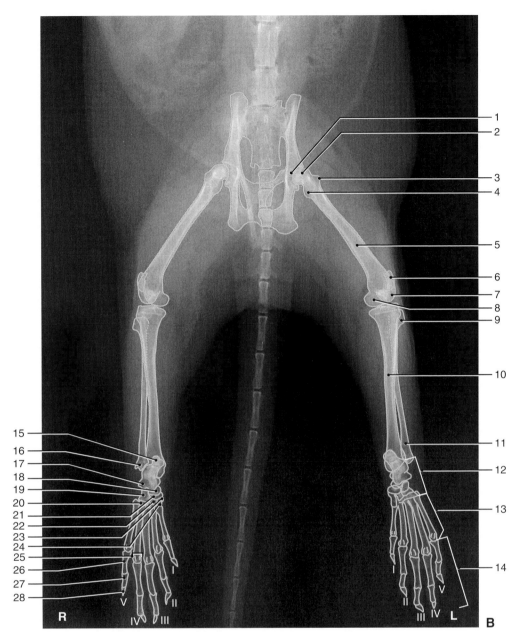

Figure 8-22, B
Type of animal: Ferret
Type of study: Pelvic limb
Projection: Ventrodorsal
Weight of animal: 1.2 kg
Gender: Male
Reproductive status: Neutered
Age: Adult

1. Acetabulum
2. Femoral head
3. Greater trochanter of femur
4. Lesser trochanter of femur
5. Femur
6. Patella
7. Lateral femoral condyle
8. Medial femoral condyle
9. Head of fibula
10. Tibia
11. Fibula
12. Tarsal bones
13. Metatarsal bones
14. Phalanges
15. Calcaneal tuber
16. Lateral malleolus of fibula
17. Calcaneus
18. Talus
19. Tarsal bone IV
20. Tarsal bone III
21. Central tarsal bone
22. Tarsal bone II
23. Tarsal bone I
24. Metatarsal bone I
25. Proximal sesamoid bones
26. Proximal phalanx of digit V
27. Middle phalanx of digit V
28. Distal phalanx of digit V

Figure 8-23, A
Type of animal: Ferret
Type of study: Stifle joint
Projection: Mediolateral
Weight of animal: 1.2 kg
Gender: Male
Reproductive status: Neutered
Age: Adult

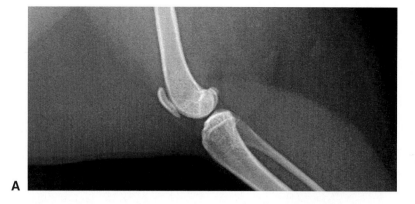

Figure 8-23, B
Type of animal: Ferret
Type of study: Stifle joint
Projection: Mediolateral
Weight of animal: 1.2 kg
Gender: Male
Reproductive status: Neutered
Age: Adult

1. Femur
2. Fabella
3. Fibula
4. Patella
5. Femoral condyle
6. Tibia

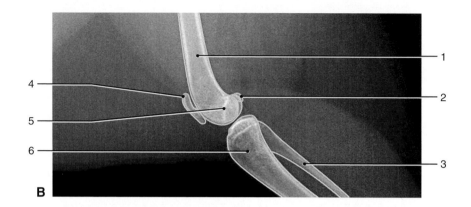

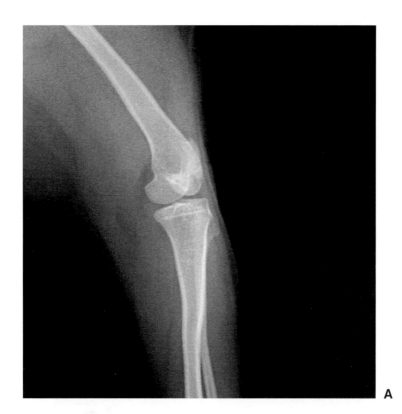

Figure 8-24, A
Type of animal: Ferret
Type of study: Stifle joint
Projection: Craniocaudal
Weight of animal: 1.2 kg
Gender: Male
Reproductive status: Neutered
Age: Adult

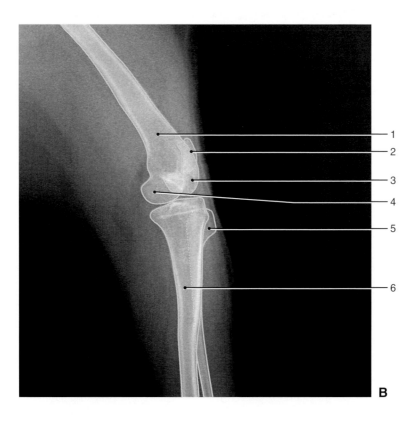

Figure 8-24, B
Type of animal: Ferret
Type of study: Stifle joint
Projection: Craniocaudal
Weight of animal: 1.2 kg
Gender: Male
Reproductive status: Neutered
Age: Adult

1. Femur
2. Patella
3. Lateral femoral condyle
4. Medial femoral condyle
5. Fibula
6. Tibia

Figure 8-25, A
Type of animal: Ferret
Type of study: Distal pelvic limb
Projection: Mediolateral
Weight of animal: 1.2 kg
Gender: Male
Reproductive status: Neutered
Age: Adult

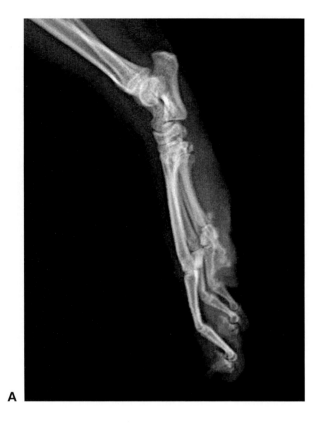

A

Figure 8-25, B
Type of animal: Ferret
Type of study: Distal pelvic limb
Projection: Mediolateral
Weight of animal: 1.2 kg
Gender: Male
Reproductive status: Neutered
Age: Adult

1. Fibula
2. Calcaneal tuber
3. Tarsal bones
4. Metatarsal bones
5. Phalanges
6. Tibia
7. Talus
8. Trochlea of talus
9. Calcaneus
10. Tarsal bone IV
11. Central tarsal bone
12. Tarsal bones I, II, and III
13. Proximal sesamoid bone
14. Metatarsal bone
15. Proximal phalanx
16. Middle phalanx
17. Distal phalanx

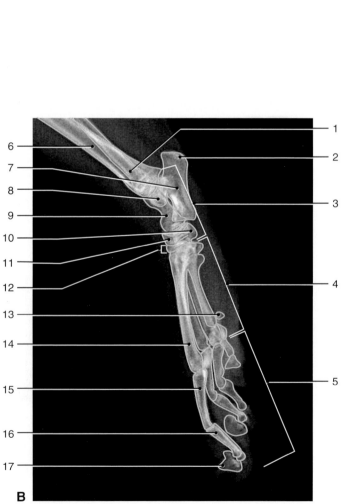

B

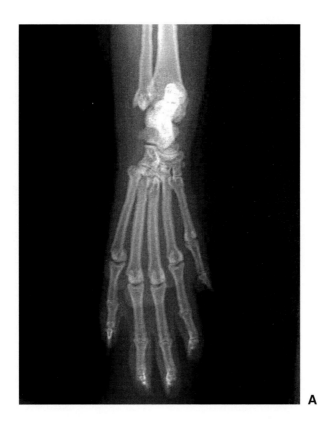

A

Figure 8-26, A
Type of animal: Ferret
Type of study: Distal pelvic limb
Projection: Dorsoplantar
Weight of animal: 1.2 kg
Gender: Male
Reproductive status: Neutered
Age: Adult

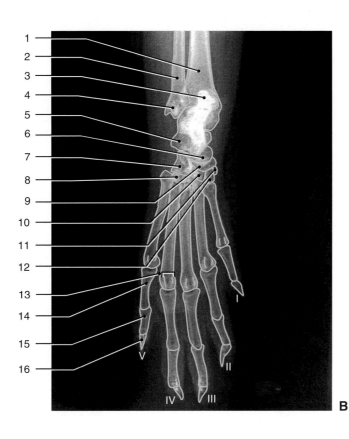

B

Figure 8-26, B
Type of animal: Ferret
Type of study: Distal pelvic limb
Projection: Dorsoplantar
Weight of animal: 1.2 kg
Gender: Male
Reproductive status: Neutered
Age: Adult

1. Tibia
2. Fibula
3. Calcaneal tuber
4. Lateral malleolus of fibula
5. Calcaneus
6. Talus
7. Tarsal bone IV
8. Tarsal bone III
9. Central tarsal bone
10. Tarsal bone II
11. Tarsal bone I
12. Metatarsal bone I
13. Proximal sesamoid bones
14. Proximal phalanx of digit V
15. Middle phalanx of digit V
16. Distal phalanx of digit V

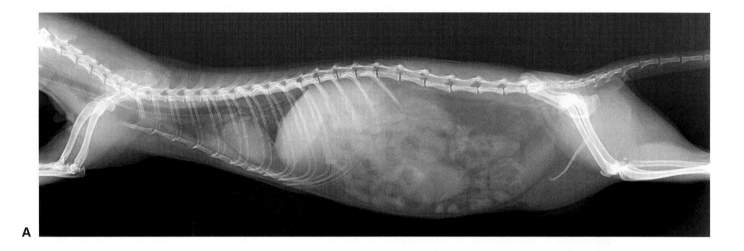

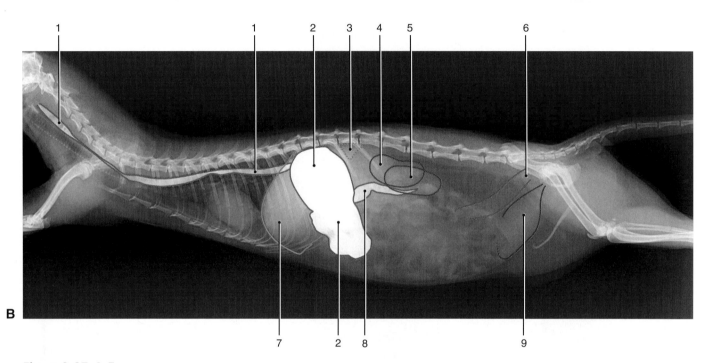

Figure 8-27, A-F

Type of animal: Ferret
Type of study: Gastrointestinal double contrast study
Contrast medium: Barium sulfate suspension (Novopaque
  60% w/v; Lafayette Pharmaceutical, Inc., Lafayette, Ind.)
  20 ml administered via esophageal gavage; 50 ml of air
  infused 30 min following contrast administration
Projection: Laterolateral
Weight of animal: 1.2 kg
Gender: Male
Reproductive status: Neutered
Age: Adult

1. Esophagus
2. Stomach
3. Spleen
4. Right kidney
5. Left kidney
6. Descending colon
7. Liver
8. Duodenum
9. Urinary bladder
10. Small intestine
11. Rectum

Image	Time (min)	Position
A	Survey	R lateral
B	1	R lateral

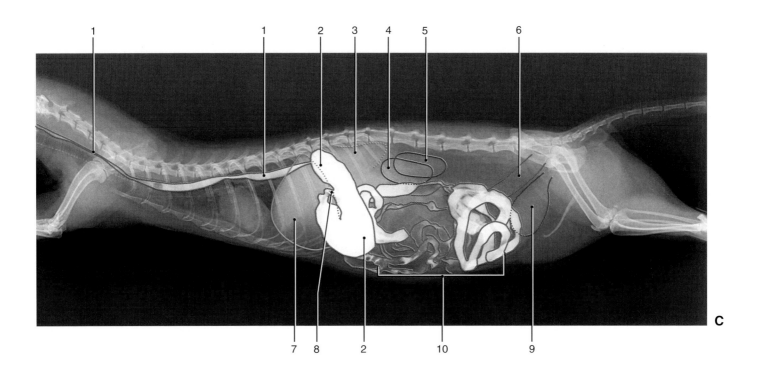

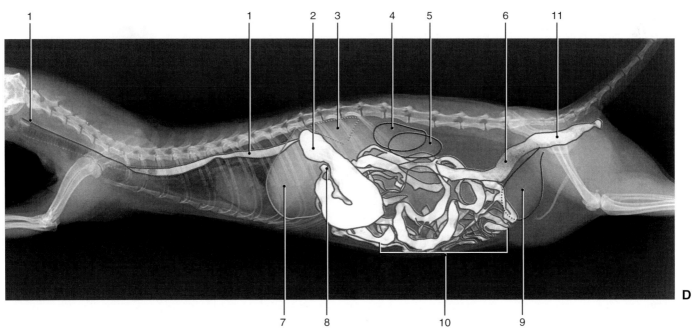

Figure 8-27, A-F—cont'd

Type of animal: Ferret
Type of study: Gastrointestinal double contrast study
Contrast medium: Barium sulfate suspension (Novopaque
  60% w/v; Lafayette Pharmaceutical, Inc., Lafayette, Ind.)
  20 ml administered via esophageal gavage; 50 ml of air
  infused 30 min following contrast administration
Projection: Laterolateral
Weight of animal: 1.2 kg
Gender: Male
Reproductive status: Neutered
Age: Adult

1. Esophagus
2. Stomach
3. Spleen
4. Right kidney
5. Left kidney
6. Descending colon
7. Liver
8. Duodenum
9. Urinary bladder
10. Small intestine
11. Rectum

Image	Time (min)	Position
C	15	R lateral
D	30*	R lateral

*50 ml of air was infused into the stomach after image D (30 min)
was obtained.

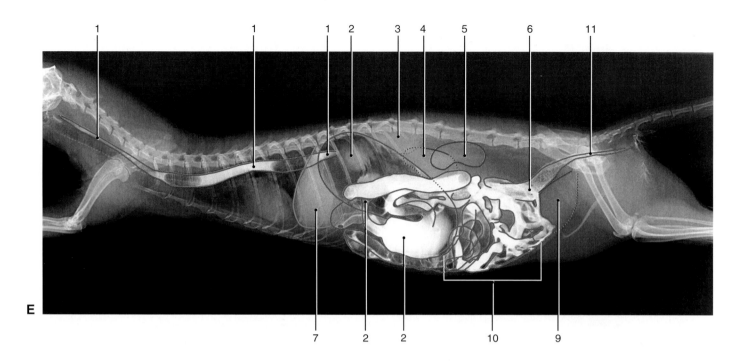

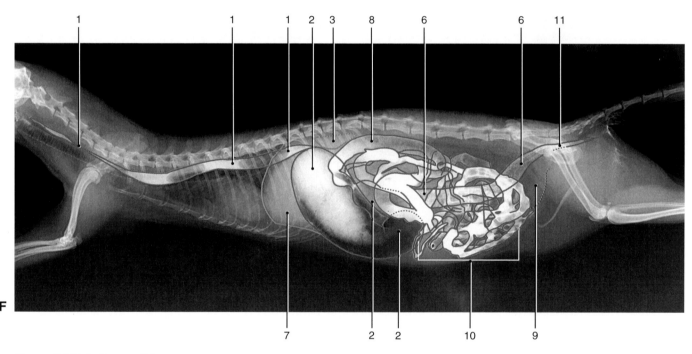

Figure 8-27, A-F—cont'd

Type of animal: Ferret

Type of study: Gastrointestinal double contrast study

Contrast medium: Barium sulfate suspension (Novopaque 60% w/v; Lafayette Pharmaceutical, Inc., Lafayette, Ind.) 20 ml administered via esophageal gavage; 50 ml of air infused 30 min following contrast administration

Projection: Laterolateral

Weight of animal: 1.2 kg

Gender: Male

Reproductive status: Neutered

Age: Adult

1. Esophagus
2. Stomach
3. Spleen
4. Right kidney
5. Left kidney
6. Descending colon
7. Liver
8. Duodenum
9. Urinary bladder
10. Small intestine
11. Rectum

Image	Time (min)	Position
E	35	R lateral
F	35	L lateral

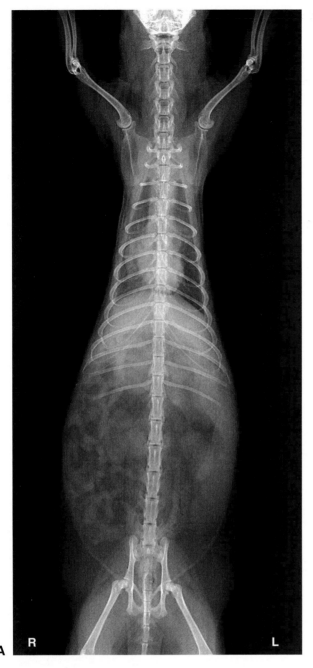

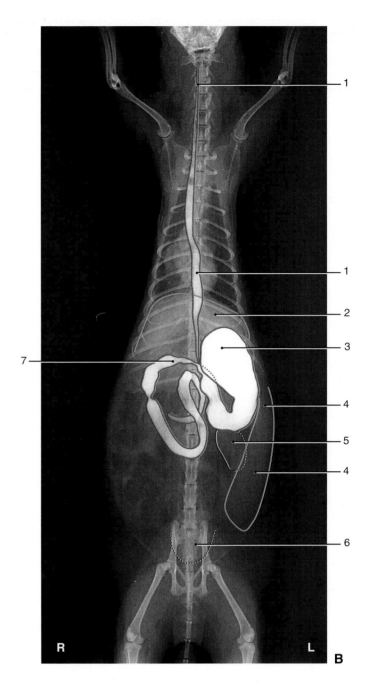

Figure 8-28, A-F
Type of animal: Ferret
Type of study: Gastrointestinal double contrast study
Contrast medium: Barium sulfate suspension (Novopaque
   60% w/v; Lafayette Pharmaceutical, Inc., Lafayette,
   Ind.) 20 ml administered via esophageal gavage; 50 ml
   of air infused 30 min following contrast administration
Projection: Ventrodorsal (except for image F)
Weight of animal: 1.2 kg
Gender: Male
Reproductive status: Neutered
Age: Adult

1. Esophagus	8. Right kidney
2. Liver	9. Small intestine
3. Stomach	10. Rectum
4. Spleen	11. Transverse colon
5. Left kidney	12. Ascending colon
6. Urinary bladder	13. Descending colon
7. Duodenum	

Image	Time (min)	Position
A	Survey	VD
B	1	VD

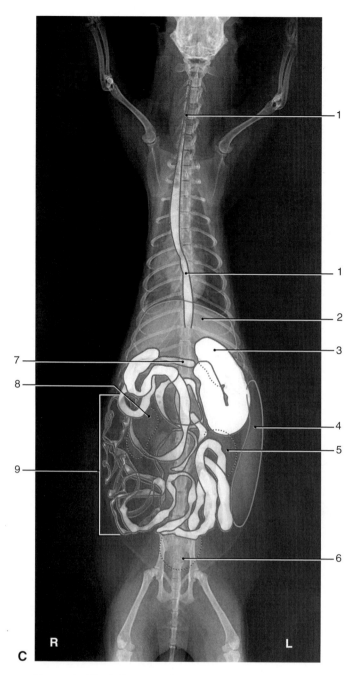

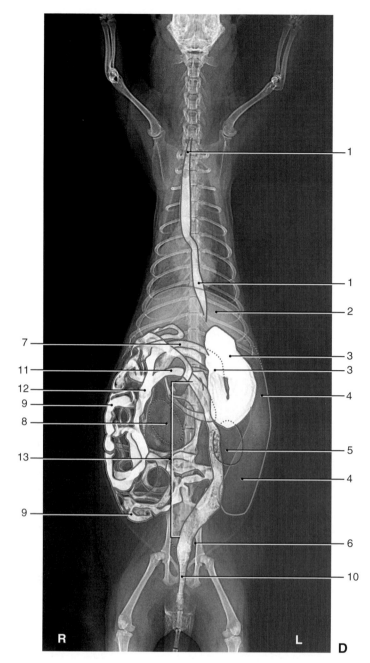

Figure 8-28, A-F—cont'd

Type of animal: Ferret

Type of study: Gastrointestinal double contrast study

Contrast medium: Barium sulfate suspension (Novopaque 60% w/v; Lafayette Pharmaceutical, Inc., Lafayette, Ind.) 20 ml administered via esophageal gavage; 50 ml of air infused 30 min following contrast administration

Projection: Ventrodorsal (except for image F)

Weight of animal: 1.2 kg

Gender: Male

Reproductive status: Neutered

Age: Adult

1.	Esophagus	8. Right kidney
2.	Liver	9. Small intestine
3.	Stomach	10. Rectum
4.	Spleen	11. Transverse colon
5.	Left kidney	12. Ascending colon
6.	Urinary bladder	13. Descending colon
7.	Duodenum	

Image	Time (min)	Position
C	15	VD
D	30*	VD

*50 ml of air was infused into the stomach after image D (30 min) was obtained.

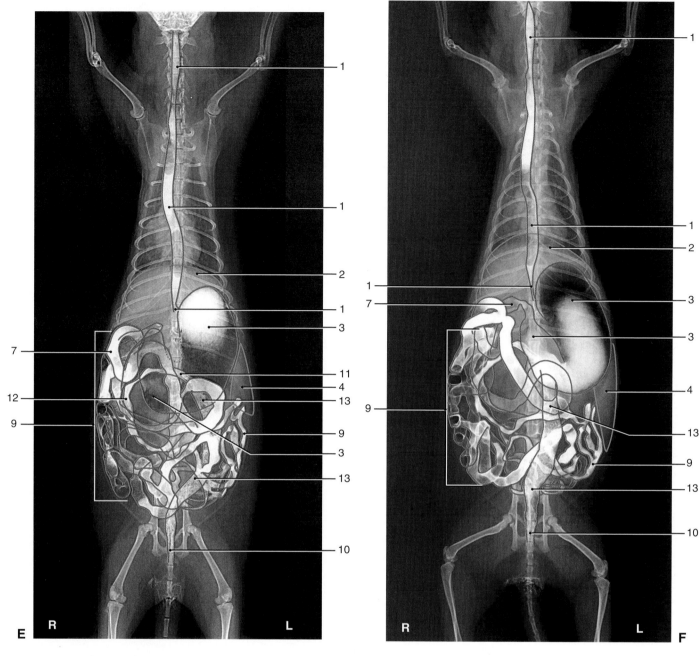

Figure 8-28, A-F—cont'd
Type of animal: Ferret
Type of study: Gastrointestinal double contrast study
Contrast medium: Barium sulfate suspension (Novopaque 60% w/v; Lafayette Pharmaceutical, Inc., Lafayette, Ind.) 20 ml administered via esophageal gavage; 50 ml of air infused 30 min following contrast administration
Projection: Ventrodorsal (except for image F)
Weight of animal: 1.2 kg
Gender: Male
Reproductive status: Neutered
Age: Adult

1. Esophagus	8. Right kidney
2. Liver	9. Small intestine
3. Stomach	10. Rectum
4. Spleen	11. Transverse colon
5. Left kidney	12. Ascending colon
6. Urinary bladder	13. Descending colon
7. Duodenum	

Image	Time (min)	Position
E	35	VD
F	35	DV

Figure 8-29, A-E
Type of animal: Ferret
Type of study: Excretory urogram
Contrast medium: RenoCal-76
   (37% organically bound
   iodine; Bracco Diagnostics, Inc.,
   Princeton, NJ) 2.75 ml IV (2.3 ml/kg)
Projection: Laterolateral
   (right lateral recumbency)
Weight of animal: 1.2 kg
Gender: Male
Reproductive status: Neutered
Age: Adult

Image	Time (min)
A	0
B	5

1. Right kidney
2. Left kidney
3. Right ureter
4. Left ureter
5. Urinary bladder
6. Renal pelvis
7. Recesses of renal pelvis
8. Compression bandage

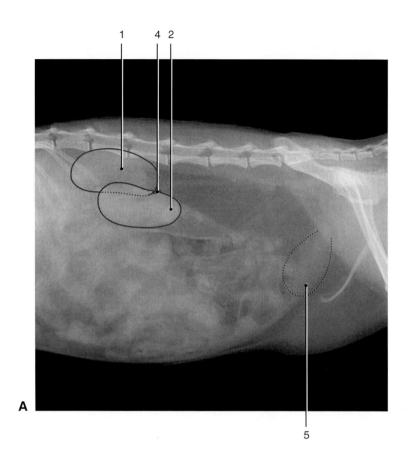

A

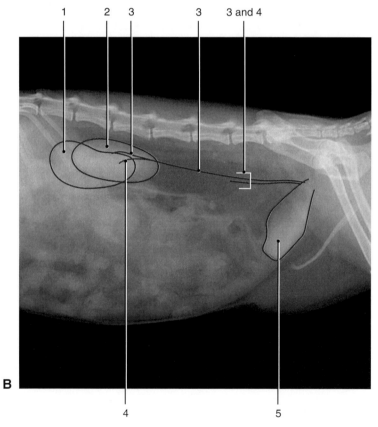

B

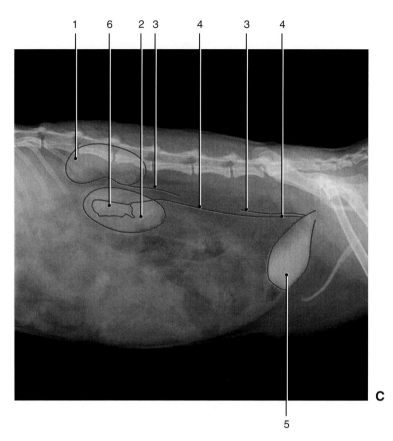

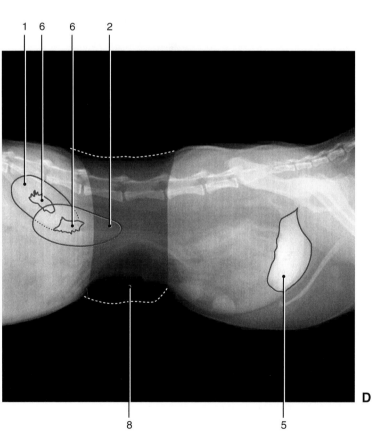

Figure 8-29, A-E—cont'd
Type of animal: Ferret
Type of study: Excretory urogram
Contrast medium: RenoCal-76
   (37% organically bound
   iodine; Bracco Diagnostics, Inc.,
   Princeton, NJ) 2.75 ml IV (2.3 ml/kg)
Projection: Laterolateral
   (right lateral recumbency)
Weight of animal: 1.2 kg
Gender: Male
Reproductive status: Neutered
Age: Adult

Image	Time (min)
C	10
D	35*

*25 min following application
of compression bandage.

1. Right kidney
2. Left kidney
3. Right ureter
4. Left ureter
5. Urinary bladder
6. Renal pelvis
7. Recesses of renal pelvis
8. Compression bandage

Figure 8-29, A-E—cont'd
Type of animal: Ferret
Type of study: Excretory urogram
Contrast medium: RenoCal-76
    (37% organically bound
    iodine; Bracco Diagnostics, Inc.,
    Princeton, NJ) 2.75 ml IV (2.3 ml/kg)
Projection: Laterolateral
    (right lateral recumbency)
Weight of animal: 1.2 kg
Gender: Male
Reproductive status: Neutered
Age: Adult

Image	Time (min)
E	60*

*25 min following release of compression bandage.

1. Right kidney
2. Left kidney
3. Right ureter
4. Left ureter
5. Urinary bladder
6. Renal pelvis
7. Recesses of renal pelvis
8. Compression bandage

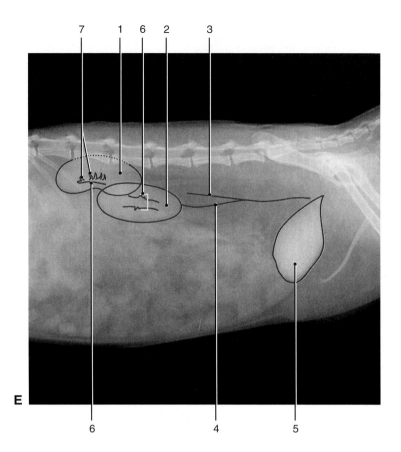

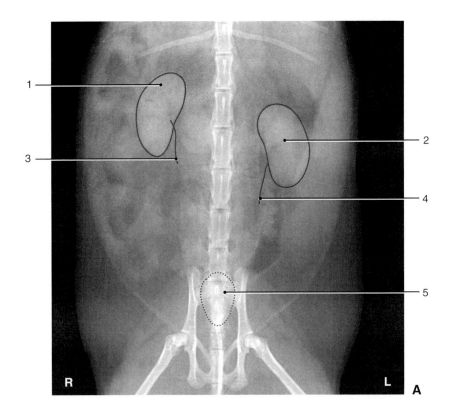

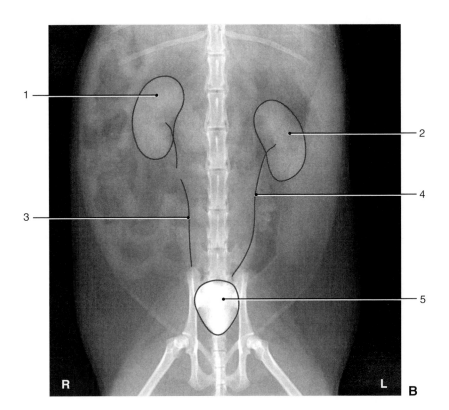

Figure 8-30, A-E
Type of animal: Ferret
Type of study: Excretory urogram
Contrast medium: RenoCal-76
   (37% organically bound
   iodine; Bracco Diagnostics, Inc.,
   Princeton, NJ) 2.75 ml IV (2.3 ml/kg)
Projection: Ventrodorsal
Weight of animal: 1.2 kg
Gender: Male
Reproductive status: Neutered
Age: Adult

Image	Time (min)
A	0
B	5

1. Right kidney
2. Left kidney
3. Right ureter
4. Left ureter
5. Urinary bladder
6. Renal pelvis
7. Recesses of renal pelvis
8. Compression bandage

Figure 8-30, A-E—cont'd
Type of animal: Ferret
Type of study: Excretory urogram
Contrast medium: RenoCal-76
   (37% organically bound
   iodine; Bracco Diagnostics, Inc.,
   Princeton, NJ) 2.75 ml IV (2.3 ml/kg)
Projection: Ventrodorsal
Weight of animal: 1.2 kg
Gender: Male
Reproductive status: Neutered
Age: Adult

Image	Time (min)
C	10
D	35*

*25 min following application
of compression bandage.

1. Right kidney
2. Left kidney
3. Right ureter
4. Left ureter
5. Urinary bladder
6. Renal pelvis
7. Recesses of renal pelvis
8. Compression bandage

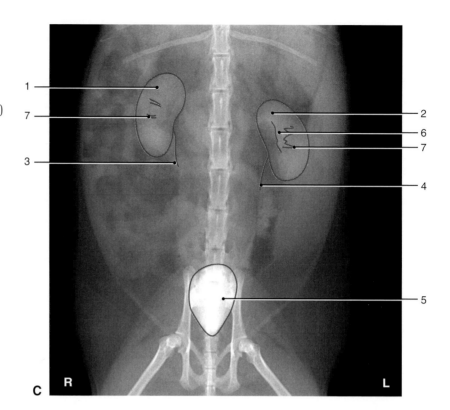

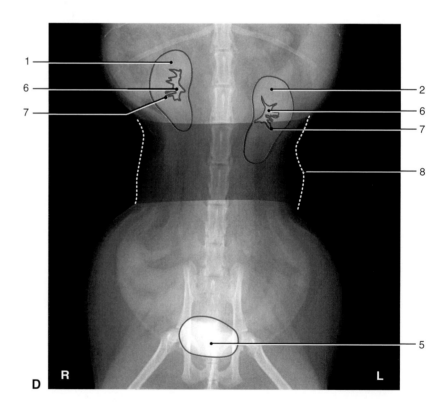

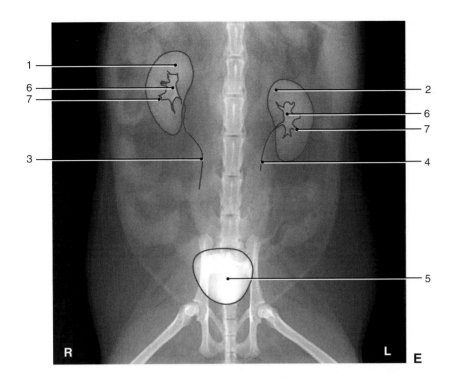

Figure 8-30, A-E—cont'd
Type of animal: Ferret
Type of study: Excretory urogram
Contrast medium: RenoCal-76
    (37% organically bound
    iodine; Bracco Diagnostics, Inc.,
    Princeton, NJ) 2.75 ml IV (2.3 ml/kg)
Projection: Ventrodorsal
Weight of animal: 1.2 kg
Gender: Male
Reproductive status: Neutered
Age: Adult

Image	Time (min)
E	60*

*25 min following release
of compression bandage.

1. Right kidney
2. Left kidney
3. Right ureter
4. Left ureter
5. Urinary bladder
6. Renal pelvis
7. Recesses of renal pelvis
8. Compression bandage

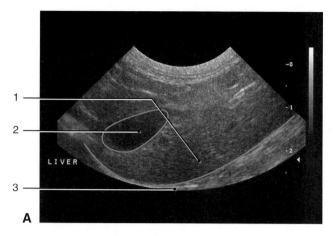

Figure 8-31, A
Transverse image of liver

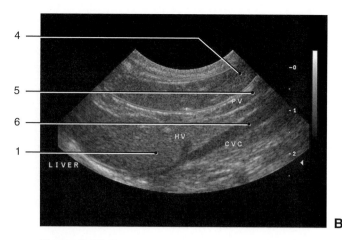

Figure 8-31, B
Sagittal image of liver*

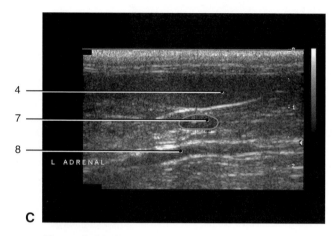

Figure 8-31, C
Sagittal image of spleen

Figure 8-31, A-C
Type of animal: Ferret
Type of study: Ultrasound study of liver and spleen
Weight of animal: 1.2 kg
Gender: Male
Reproductive status: Neutered
Age: Adult

1. Liver
2. Gallbladder
3. Diaphragm
4. Spleen
5. Portal vein
6. Caudal vena cava
7. Left adrenal gland
8. Aorta

*CVC, Caudal vena cava; HV, hepatic vein; PV, portal vein.

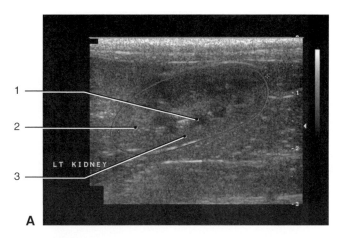

Figure 8-32, A
Sagittal image of left kidney

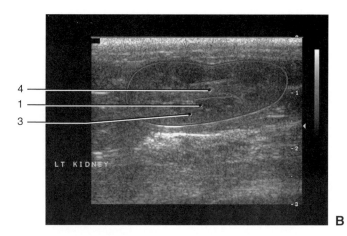

Figure 8-32, B
Sagittal image of left kidney

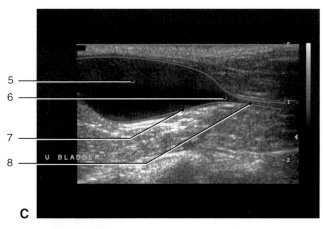

Figure 8-32, C
Sagittal image of urinary bladder

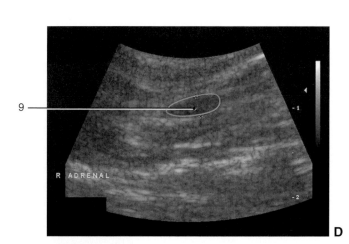

Figure 8-32, D
Sagittal image of right adrenal gland

Figure 8-32, A-D
Type of animal: Ferret
Type of study: Ultrasound study of urinary tract and associated
    structures
Weight of animal: 1.2 kg
Gender: Male
Reproductive status: Neutered
Age: Adult

1. Renal medulla
2. Cranial pole of left kidney
3. Renal cortex
4. Renal pelvis
5. Body of urinary bladder
6. Neck of urinary bladder
7. Wall of urinary bladder
8. Urethra
9. Right adrenal gland

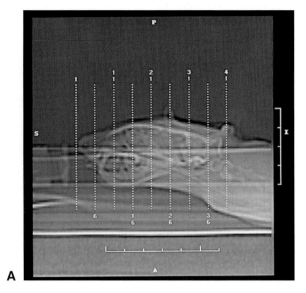

A

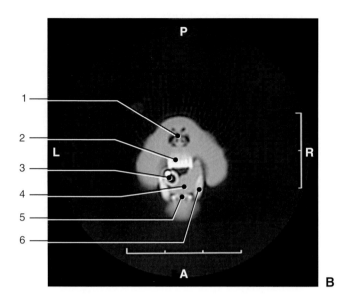

B

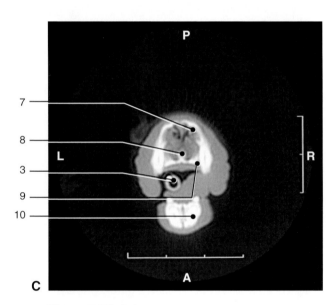

C

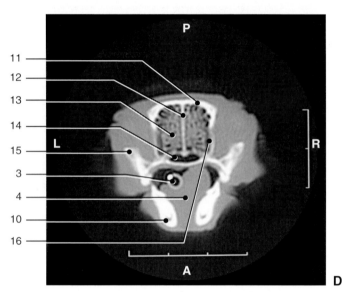

D

Figure 8-33, A-L

Type of animal: Ferret
Type of study: CT head
Imaging plane: Transverse
Weight of animal: 1.2 kg
Gender: Male
Reproductive status: Neutered
Age: Adult

1. External nare
2. Maxillary incisor tooth
3. Endotracheal tube
4. Tongue
5. Mandibular incisor tooth
6. Maxillary canine tooth
7. Nasal cavity
8. Vomer
9. Palatine bone
10. Mandible
11. Nasal bone
12. Nasal septum
13. Nasoturbinates
14. Nasopharynx
15. Zygomatic bone
16. Maxilla
17. Ethmoturbinates

18. Cerebrum
19. Sphenopalatine sinus
20. Frontal sinus
21. Pterygoid bone
22. Sella turcica
23. Tympanic cavity
24. Petrous part of temporal bone
25. Ear canal
26. Hyoid bone
27. Sagittal crest
28. Tentorium cerebelli osseum
29. Inner ears
30. Occipital bone
31. Foramen magnum
32. Occipital condyle
33. Atlas

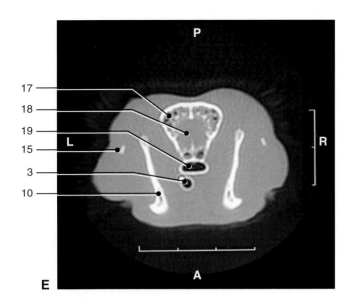

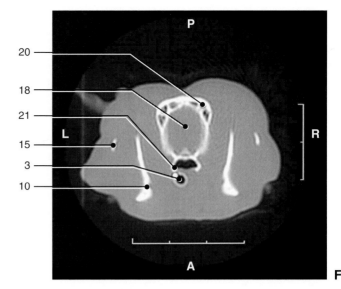

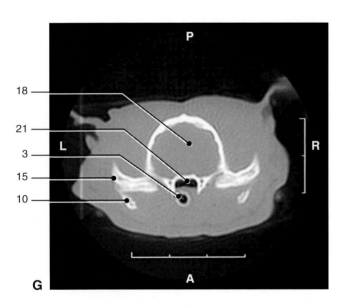

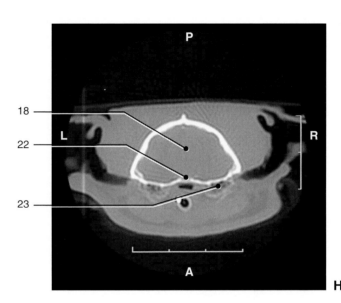

Figure 8-33, A-L—cont'd
Type of animal: Ferret
Type of study: CT head
Imaging plane: Transverse
Weight of animal: 1.2 kg
Gender: Male
Reproductive status: Neutered
Age: Adult

1. External nare
2. Maxillary incisor tooth
3. Endotracheal tube
4. Tongue
5. Mandibular incisor tooth
6. Maxillary canine tooth
7. Nasal cavity
8. Vomer
9. Palatine bone
10. Mandible
11. Nasal bone
12. Nasal septum
13. Nasoturbinates
14. Nasopharynx
15. Zygomatic bone
16. Maxilla
17. Ethmoturbinates

18. Cerebrum
19. Sphenopalatine sinus
20. Frontal sinus
21. Pterygoid bone
22. Sella turcica
23. Tympanic cavity
24. Petrous part of temporal bone
25. Ear canal
26. Hyoid bone
27. Sagittal crest
28. Tentorium cerebelli osseum
29. Inner ears
30. Occipital bone
31. Foramen magnum
32. Occipital condyle
33. Atlas

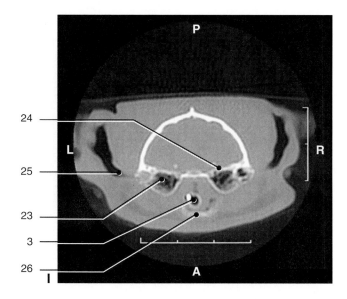

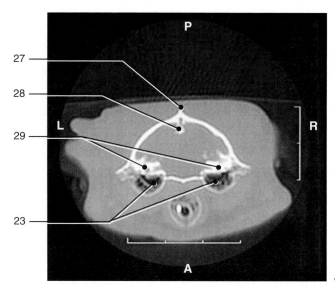

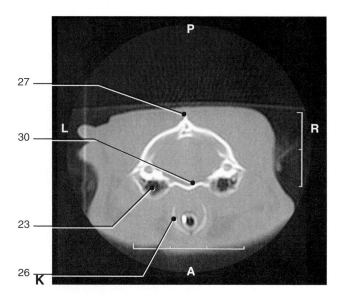

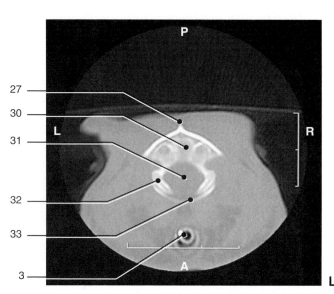

Figure 8-33, A-L—cont'd
Type of animal: Ferret
Type of study: CT head
Imaging plane: Transverse
Weight of animal: 1.2 kg
Gender: Male
Reproductive status: Neutered
Age: Adult

1. External nare
2. Maxillary incisor tooth
3. Endotracheal tube
4. Tongue
5. Mandibular incisor tooth
6. Maxillary canine tooth
7. Nasal cavity
8. Vomer
9. Palatine bone
10. Mandible
11. Nasal bone
12. Nasal septum
13. Nasoturbinates
14. Nasopharynx
15. Zygomatic bone
16. Maxilla
17. Ethmoturbinates

18. Cerebrum
19. Sphenopalatine sinus
20. Frontal sinus
21. Pterygoid bone
22. Sella turcica
23. Tympanic cavity
24. Petrous part of temporal bone
25. Ear canal
26. Hyoid bone
27. Sagittal crest
28. Tentorium cerebelli osseum
29. Inner ears
30. Occipital bone
31. Foramen magnum
32. Occipital condyle
33. Atlas

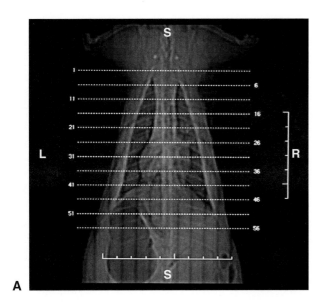

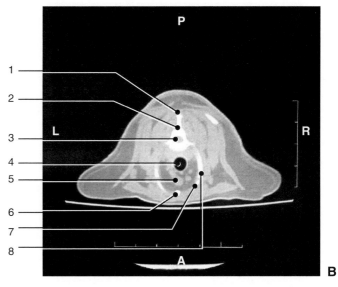

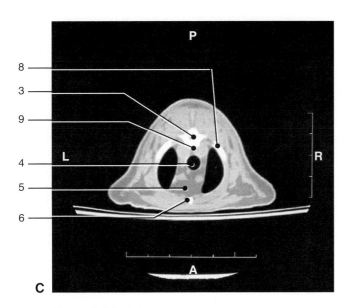

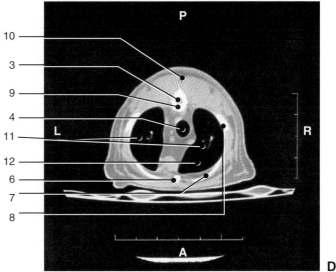

Figure 8-34, A-J

Type of animal: Ferret
Type of study: CT thorax
Imaging plane: Transverse
Weight of animal: 1.2 kg
Gender: Male
Reproductive status: Neutered
Age: Adult

1. Spinous process of thoracic vertebra
2. Dorsal lamina of thoracic vertebra
3. Spinal canal of thoracic vertebra
4. Trachea
5. Cranial mediastinum
6. Sternebra
7. Costochondral joint
8. Rib
9. Thoracic vertebra
10. Epaxial muscles
11. Pulmonary vasculature
12. Lung
13. Bronchi
14. Left ventricle of heart
15. Carina of trachea
16. Pericardial adipose tissue
17. Caudal mediastinum
18. Liver
19. Fundus of stomach
20. Spleen
21. Falciform adipose tissue

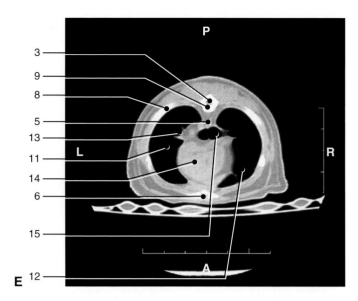

E

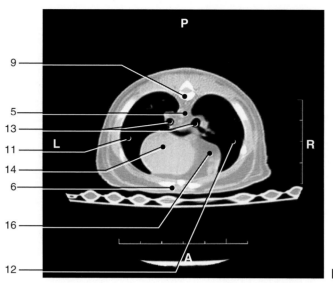

F

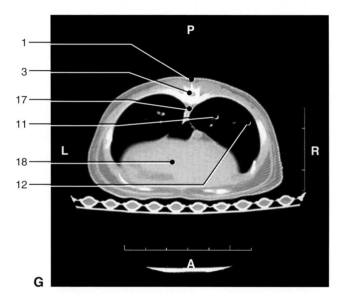

G

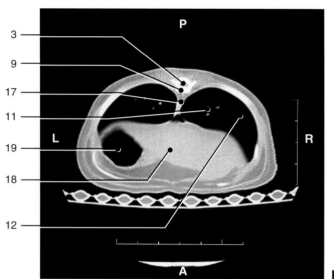

H

Figure 8-34, A-J—cont'd

Type of animal: Ferret
Type of study: CT thorax
Imaging plane: Transverse
Weight of animal: 1.2 kg
Gender: Male
Reproductive status: Neutered
Age: Adult

1. Spinous process of thoracic vertebra
2. Dorsal lamina of thoracic vertebra
3. Spinal canal of thoracic vertebra
4. Trachea
5. Cranial mediastinum
6. Sternebra
7. Costochondral joint
8. Rib
9. Thoracic vertebra
10. Epaxial muscles
11. Pulmonary vasculature

12. Lung
13. Bronchi
14. Left ventricle of heart
15. Carina of trachea
16. Pericardial adipose tissue
17. Caudal mediastinum
18. Liver
19. Fundus of stomach
20. Spleen
21. Falciform adipose tissue

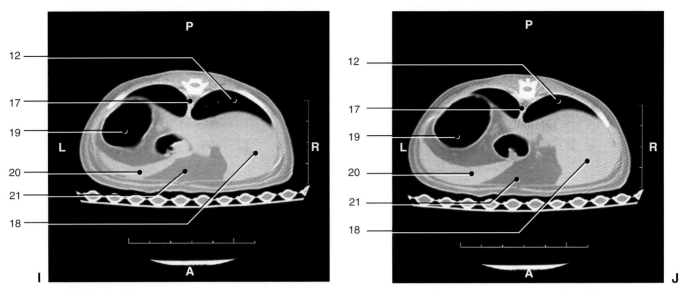

Figure 8-34, A-J—cont'd
Type of animal: Ferret
Type of study: CT thorax
Imaging plane: Transverse
Weight of animal: 1.2 kg
Gender: Male
Reproductive status: Neutered
Age: Adult

1. Spinous process of thoracic vertebra
2. Dorsal lamina of thoracic vertebra
3. Spinal canal of thoracic vertebra
4. Trachea
5. Cranial mediastinum
6. Sternebra
7. Costochondral joint
8. Rib
9. Thoracic vertebra
10. Epaxial muscles
11. Pulmonary vasculature

12. Lung
13. Bronchi
14. Left ventricle of heart
15. Carina of trachea
16. Pericardial adipose tissue
17. Caudal mediastinum
18. Liver
19. Fundus of stomach
20. Spleen
21. Falciform adipose tissue

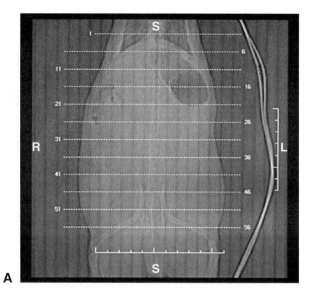

A

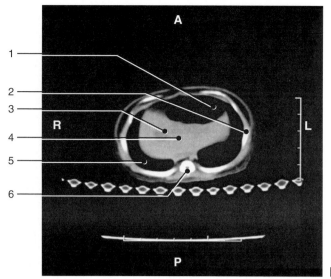

B

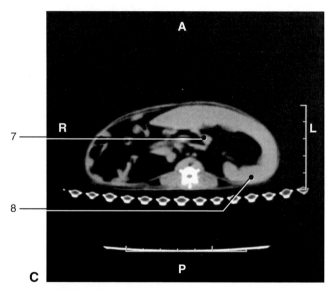

C

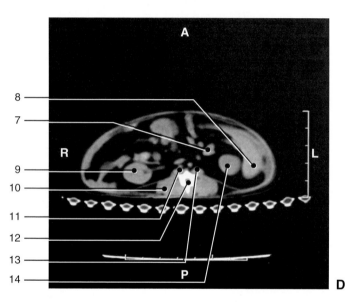

D

Figure 8-35, A-F

Type of animal: Ferret
Type of study: CT abdomen
Imaging plane: Transverse
Weight of animal: 1.2 kg
Gender: Male
Reproductive status: Neutered
Age: Adult

1. Stomach
2. Rib
3. Gallbladder
4. Liver
5. Lung
6. Thoracic vertebra
7. Intestine
8. Spleen
9. Right kidney
10. Epaxial muscles
11. Caudal vena cava

12. Lumbar vertebra
13. Aorta
14. Left kidney
15. Os penis
16. Urinary bladder
17. Colon
18. Sacral vertebra
19. Ilium
20. Pubis
21. Sacrum
22. Femur

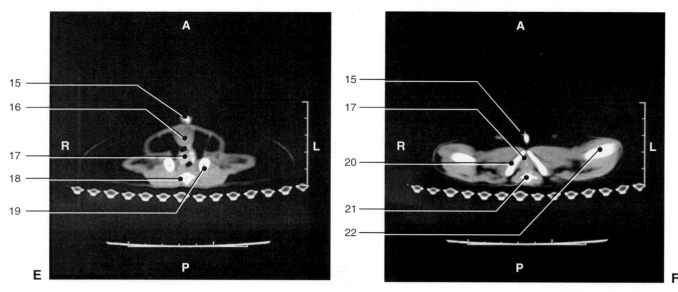

Figure 8-35, A-F—cont'd
Type of animal: Ferret
Type of study: CT abdomen
Imaging plane: Transverse
Weight of animal: 1.2 kg
Gender: Male
Reproductive status: Neutered
Age: Adult

1. Stomach
2. Rib
3. Gallbladder
4. Liver
5. Lung
6. Thoracic vertebra
7. Intestine
8. Spleen
9. Right kidney
10. Epaxial muscles
11. Caudal vena cava
12. Lumbar vertebra
13. Aorta
14. Left kidney
15. Os penis
16. Urinary bladder
17. Colon
18. Sacral vertebra
19. Ilium
20. Pubis
21. Sacrum
22. Femur

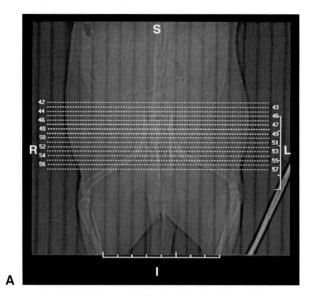

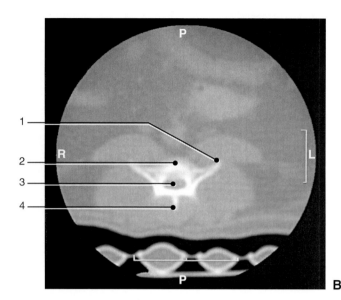

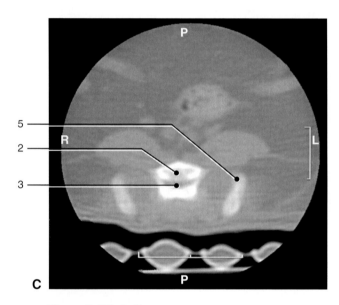

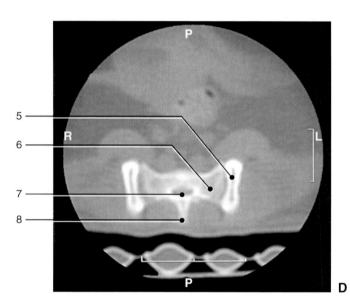

Figure 8-36, A-G

Type of animal: Ferret
Type of study: CT pelvis
Imaging plane: Transverse
Weight of animal: 1.2 kg
Gender: Male
Reproductive status: Neutered
Age: Adult

1. Transverse process of lumbar vertebra
2. Lumbar vertebra
3. Spinal canal of lumbar vertebra
4. Spinous process of lumbar vertebra
5. Ilium
6. Sacrum
7. Spinal canal of sacral vertebra
8. Spinous process of sacral vertebra
9. Colon

10. Os penis
11. Femoral head
12. Pubis
13. Acetabulum
14. Lunate surface of acetabulum
15. Greater trochanter of femur
16. Pubic symphysis
17. Caudal vertebra

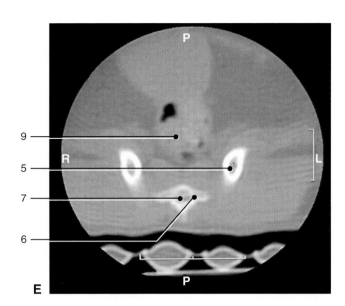

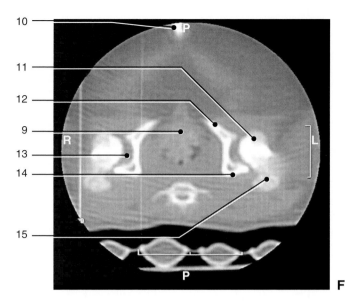

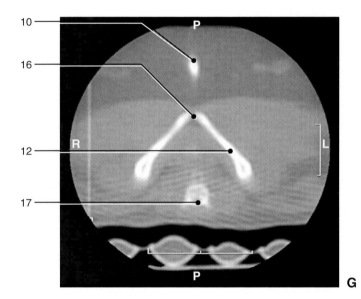

Figure 8-36, A-G—cont'd

Type of animal: Ferret
Type of study: CT pelvis
Imaging plane: Transverse
Weight of animal: 1.2 kg
Gender: Male
Reproductive status: Neutered
Age: Adult

1. Transverse process of lumbar vertebra
2. Lumbar vertebra
3. Spinal canal of lumbar vertebra
4. Spinous process of lumbar vertebra
5. Ilium
6. Sacrum
7. Spinal canal of sacral vertebra
8. Spinous process of sacral vertebra
9. Colon

10. Os penis
11. Femoral head
12. Pubis
13. Acetabulum
14. Lunate surface of acetabulum
15. Greater trochanter of femur
16. Pubic symphysis
17. Caudal vertebra

INDEX

Page numbers followed by f indicate figures; by t, tables.